# Underground Clinical Vignettes

## *Internal Medicine I*

### FOURTH EDITION

# Underground Clinical Vignettes

## Internal Medicine I

### FOURTH EDITION

**Sandra I. Kim, M.D., Ph.D.**
*Resident in Internal Medicine*
*Beth Israel Deaconess Medical Center*
*Harvard Medical School*
*Boston, Massachusetts*

**Todd A. Swanson, M.D., Ph.D.**
*Resident in Radiation Oncology*
*William Beaumont Hospital*
*Royal Oak, Michigan*

Wolters Kluwer | Lippincott Williams & Wilkins
Health
Philadelphia · Baltimore · New York · London
Buenos Aires · Hong Kong · Sydney · Tokyo

*Acquisitions Editor:* Nancy Anastasi Duffy
*Developmental Editor:* Nancy Hoffmann
*Managing Editor:* Kelly Horvath
*Associate Production Manager:* Kevin Johnson
*Marketing Manager:* Jennifer Kuklinski
*Creative Director:* Doug Smock
*Compositor:* International Typesetting and Composition

© 2007 by Lippincott Williams & Wilkins
UCV Step 2 *Internal Medicine I*, Fourth Edition

Lippincott Williams & Wilkins, a Wolters Kluwer business.

| | |
|---|---|
| 351 West Camden Street | 530 Walnut Street |
| Baltimore, MD 21201 | Philadelphia, PA 19106 |

9  8  7  6  5  4  3  2  1

**Library of Congress Cataloging-in-Publication Data**

Kim, Sandra.
    Internal medicine I.—4th ed. / Sandra I. Kim, Todd A. Swanson.
        p. ; cm.—(Underground clinical vignettes. Step 2)
    Includes index.
    Rev. ed. of: Internal medicine / Vikhas Bhushan . . . [et al.]. 3rd ed. c2005.
    ISBN-13: 978-0-7817-6835-1
    ISBN-10: 0-7817-6835-7
    1. Internal medicine—Case studies.   2. Physicians—Licenses—United States—Examinations—Study guides.  I. Swanson, Todd A.  II. Title.  III. Title: Internal medicine one.  IV. Title: Internal medicine 1.
V. Series.
    [DNLM:   1. Internal Medicine—Problems and Exercises.  WB 18.2 K49i 2007]
    RC66.I576 2007
    616—dc22

                            2007035305

DISCLAIMER

Care has been taken to confirm the accuracy of the information present and to describe generally accepted practices. However, the authors, editors, and publisher are not responsible for errors or omissions or for any consequences from application of the information in this book and make no warranty, expressed or implied, with respect to the currency, completeness, or accuracy of the contents of the publication. Application of this information in a particular situation remains the professional responsibility of the practitioner; the clinical treatments described and recommended may not be considered absolute and universal recommendations.

The authors, editors, and publisher have exerted every effort to ensure that drug selection and dosage set forth in this text are in accordance with the current recommendations and practice at the time of publication. However, in view of ongoing research, changes in government regulations, and the constant flow of information relating to drug therapy and drug reactions, the reader is urged to check the package insert for each drug for any change in indications and dosage and for added warnings and precautions. This is particularly important when the recommended agent is a new or infrequently employed drug.

Some drugs and medical devices presented in this publication have Food and Drug Administration (FDA) clearance for limited use in restricted research settings. It is the responsibility of the health care provider to ascertain the FDA status of each drug or device planned for use in their clinical practice.

To purchase additional copies of this book, call our customer service department at **(800) 638-3030** or fax orders to **(301) 223-2320**. International customers should call **(301) 223-2300**.

Visit Lippincott Williams & Wilkins on the Internet: http://www.lww.com. Lippincott Williams & Wilkins customer service representatives are available from 8:30 am to 6:00 pm, EST.

# dedication

Dedicated to the patients we care for.

# preface

First published in 1999, the Underground Clinical Vignettes series has provided thousands of students with a highly effective review tool as they prepare for medical exams, particularly the USMLE Step 1 and 2 exams. Designed as a quick study guide, each UCV book contains patient-centered clinical cases that highlight a range of medical diagnoses.

With this new edition of Step 2 Underground Clinical Vignettes, we have incorporated feedback from medical students across the country to provide updated cases with expanded treatment and discussion sections. Every title has more cases, drawing from a broader area within each discipline. A new two-page format enables readers to formulate an initial diagnosis prior to reading the answer to each case. The inclusion of relevant MRI images, x-rays, and photographs allows students to more readily visualize the physical presentation of each case. Breakout boxes, tables, and algorithms have been added, along with 20 all-new, Board-format QAs, making this edition of UCV an ideal source of information for exam review, classroom discussion, and clinical rotations.

The clinical vignettes in this Step 2 series have been revised and updated to reflect current medical thinking on medication, pathogenesis, epidemiology, management, and complications. Although each case presents most of the signs, symptoms, and diagnostic findings for a particular illness, patients typically will not present with such a "complete" picture either clinically or on a medical examination. Cases are not meant to simulate a potential real patient or an exam vignette.

Access to LWW's online companion site, ThePoint, will be offered as a premium with the purchase of the Underground Clinical Vignettes Step 2 bundle. Benefits include an online test link and 160 additional new Board-format questions covering all UCV subject areas.

We hope you will find the Underground Clinical Vignettes series informative and useful. We welcome any feedback, suggestions, or corrections you have about this series. Please contact us at LWW.com/medstudent.

# contributors

## Series Editors

**Sandra I. Kim, M.D., Ph.D.**
Resident in Internal Medicine
Beth Israel Deaconess Medical Center
Harvard Medical School
Boston, Massachusetts

**Todd A. Swanson, M.D., Ph.D.**
Resident in Radiation Oncology
William Beaumont Hospital
Royal Oak, Michigan

## Contributing Editors

**Anita Vanka, M.D.**
Resident in Internal Medicine
Beth Israel Deaconess Medical Center
Harvard Medical School
Boston, Massachusetts

**Suzelle Luc, M.D., M.P.H.**
Resident in Internal Medicine
Beth Israel Deaconess Medical Center
Harvard Medical School
Boston, Massachusetts

## Internal Medicine I Contributors

**Kelly Bodio, M.D.**
**Priya Roy, M.D.**
**Carolina Abuelo, M.D., D.T.M.&H.**
**Larissa Bornikova, M.D.**
**Claudia Denkinger, M.D., Ph.D.**
**Brian Hyett, M.D.**
**Rahul Jhaveri, M.D.**
**Pamela D. Vohra, M.D.**
**Pablo Quintero-Pinzon, M.D.**
**Erika Summers, M.D.**
**Shoshana J. Herzig, M.D.**

Meghan Delaney, M.D.
Laura Fanning, M.D.
Joseph Hardman, M.D.
Pamela Ann Jackson, M.D.
Jorge Magallon, M.D.
Connie Tsao, M.D., Ph.D.
Dan Tsyvine, M.D.

# acknowledgments

Our great thanks to the house staff and faculty from Beth Israel Deaconess, Massachusetts General Hospital, Brigham and Women's, and Children's Hospital in Boston, whose clinical cases, revisions, and suggestions were indispensable to this series.

Thanks to the editors at Lippincott, especially Nancy Hoffmann, who worked overtime on these books.

⊙

# abbreviations

| | |
|---|---|
| A-a | alveolar-arterial (oxygen gradient) |
| AAA | abdominal aortic aneurysm |
| ABCs | airway, breathing, circulation |
| ABGs | arterial blood gases |
| ABPA | allergic bronchopulmonary aspergillosis |
| ABVD | Adriamycin, bleomycin, vinblastine, dacarbazine (chemotherapy) |
| ACE | angiotensin-converting enzyme |
| ACTH | adrenocorticotropic hormone |
| ADA | adenosine deaminase; American Diabetic Association |
| ADH | antidiuretic hormone |
| ADHD | attention-deficit hyperactivity disorder |
| AED | automatic external defibrillator |
| AFP | $\alpha$-fetoprotein |
| AI | aortic insufficiency |
| AICD | automatic internal cardiac defibrillator |
| AIDS | acquired immunodeficiency syndrome |
| ALL | acute lymphocytic leukemia |
| ALS | amyotrophic lateral sclerosis |
| ALT | alanine aminotransferase |
| AML | acute myelogenous leukemia |
| AMP | adenosine monophosphate |
| ANA | antinuclear antibody |
| ANCA | antineutrophil cytoplasmic antibody |
| Angio | angiography |
| AP | anteroposterior |
| aPTT | activated partial thromboplastin time |
| ARDS | adult respiratory distress syndrome |
| ARF | acute renal failure |
| AS | ankylosing spondylitis |
| ASA | acetylsalicylic acid |
| 5-ASA | 5-aminosalicylic acid |
| ASD | atrial septal defect |
| ASO | antistreptolysin O |
| AST | aspartate aminotransferase |
| ATLS | Advanced Trauma Life Support (protocol) |
| ATN | acute tubular necrosis |
| ATPase | adenosine triphosphatase |
| ATRA | *all-trans*-retinoic acid |
| AV | arteriovenous, atrioventricular |
| AVPD | avoidant personality disorder |
| AXR | abdominal x-ray |
| AZT | azidothymidine (zidovudine) |
| BCG | bacille Calmette-Guérin |
| BE | barium enema |
| BP | blood pressure |
| BPD | borderline personality disorder |
| BPH | benign prostatic hypertrophy |
| BPK | B-cell progenitor kinase |
| BPM | beats per minute |
| BUN | blood urea nitrogen |
| CAA | cerebral amyloid angiopathy |
| CABG | coronary artery bypass grafting |
| CAD | coronary artery disease |
| CALLA | common acute lymphoblastic leukemia antigen |
| C-ANCA | cytoplasmic antineutrophil cytoplasmic antibody |
| CAO | chronic airway obstruction |
| CAP | community-acquired pneumonia |
| CBC | complete blood count |
| CBD | common bile duct |
| CBT | cognitive behavioral therapy |
| CCU | cardiac care unit |
| CD | cluster of differentiation |
| CDC | Centers for Disease Control |
| CEA | carcinoembryonic antigen |
| CF | cystic fibrosis |
| CFTR | cystic fibrosis transmembrane regulator |
| CFU | colony-forming unit |
| CHF | congestive heart failure |
| CJD | Creutzfeldt–Jakob disease |
| CK | creatine kinase |
| CK-MB | creatine kinase, MB fraction |
| CLL | chronic lymphocytic leukemia |
| CML | chronic myelogenous leukemia |

| | | | | |
|---|---|---|---|---|
| CMV | cytomegalovirus | | EMG | electromyography |
| CN | cranial nerve | | ER | emergency room |
| CNS | central nervous system | | ERCP | endoscopic retrograde |
| CO | cardiac output | | | cholangiopancreatography |
| COPD | chronic obstructive pulmonary | | ESR | erythrocyte sedimentation rate |
| | disease | | EtOH | ethanol |
| CPAP | continuous positive airway | | FDA | Food and Drug Administration |
| | pressure | | $Fe_{Na}$ | fractional excretion of sodium |
| CPK | creatine phosphokinase | | $FEV_1$ | forced expiratory volume in |
| CPR | cardiopulmonary resuscitation | | | 1 second |
| CRP | C-reactive protein | | FIGO | International Federation of |
| CSF | cerebrospinal fluid | | | Gynecology and Obstetrics |
| CT | computed tomography | | | (classification) |
| CVA | cerebrovascular accident | | $FIo_2$ | fraction of inspired oxygen |
| CXR | chest x-ray | | FNA | fine-needle aspiration |
| D&C | dilatation and curettage | | FRC | functional residual capacity |
| DAF | decay-accelerating factor | | FSH | follicle-stimulating hormone |
| DC | direct current | | FTA | fluorescent treponemal antibody |
| DEXA | dual-energy x-ray absorptiometry | | FTA-ABS | fluorescent treponemal antibody |
| DHEA | dehydroepiandrosterone | | | absorption test |
| DIC | disseminated intravascular | | 5-FU | 5-fluorouracil |
| | coagulation | | FVC | forced vital capacity |
| DIP | distal interphalangeal (joint) | | G6PD | glucose-6-phosphate |
| DKA | diabetic ketoacidosis | | | dehydrogenase |
| $DL_{CO}$ | diffusing capacity of carbon | | GA | gestational age |
| | monoxide | | GABA | gamma-aminobutyric acid |
| DM | diabetes mellitus | | GABHS | group A β-hemolytic |
| DMD | Duchenne muscular dystrophy | | | streptococcus |
| DNA | deoxyribonucleic acid | | GAD | generalized anxiety disorder |
| DNase | deoxyribonuclease | | GBM | glomerular basement membrane |
| dsDNA | double-stranded DNA | | G-CSF | granulocyte colony-stimulating |
| DTP | diphtheria, tetanus, pertussis | | | factor |
| | (vaccine) | | GERD | gastroesophageal reflux disease |
| DTRs | deep tendon reflexes | | GFR | glomerular filtration rate |
| DTs | delirium tremens | | GGT | gamma-glutamyltransferase |
| DUB | dysfunctional uterine bleeding | | GI | gastrointestinal |
| DVT | deep venous thrombosis | | GnRH | gonadotropin-releasing hormone |
| EBV | Epstein–Barr virus | | GU | genitourinary |
| ECG | electrocardiography | | HAV | hepatitis A virus |
| Echo | echocardiography | | Hb | hemoglobin |
| ECMO | extracorporeal membrane | | HBcAg | hepatitis B core antigen |
| | oxygenation | | HBsAg | hepatitis B surface antigen |
| EDTA | ethylenediamine tetraacetic acid | | HBV | hepatitis B virus |
| EEG | electroencephalography | | hCG | human chorionic gonadotropin |
| EF | ejection fraction | | HCl | hydrogen chloride |
| EGD | esophagogastroduodenoscopy | | $HCO_3$ | bicarbonate |
| E:I | expiratory-to-inspiratory (ratio) | | Hct | hematocrit |
| ELISA | enzyme-linked immunosorbent | | HCV | hepatitis C virus |
| | assay | | HDL | high-density lipoprotein |
| EM | electron microscopy | | HEENT | head, eyes, ears, nose, and throat |

| | | | |
|---|---|---|---|
| HELLP | hemolysis, elevated liver enzymes, low platelets (syndrome) | KUB | kidney, ureter, bladder |
| | | LA | left atrium |
| HEV | hepatitis E virus | LAMB | lentigines, atrial myxoma, blue nevi (syndrome) |
| HGPRT | hypoxanthine-guanine phosphoribosyltransferase | LD | Leishman–Donovan (body) |
| HHV | human herpesvirus | LDH | lactate dehydrogenase |
| 5-HIAA | 5-hydroxyindoleacetic acid | LDL | low-density lipoprotein |
| HIDA | hepato-iminodiacetic acid (scan) | LES | lower esophageal sphincter |
| HIV | human immunodeficiency virus | LFTs | liver function tests |
| HLA | human leukocyte antigen | LH | luteinizing hormone |
| HPF | high-power field | LHRH | luteinizing hormone–releasing hormone |
| HPI | history of present illness | | |
| HPV | human papillomavirus | LKM | liver-kidney microsomal (antibody) |
| HR | heart rate | LMN | lower motor neuron |
| HRCT | high-resolution computed tomography | LP | lumbar puncture |
| | | L/S | lecithin-to-sphingomyelin (ratio) |
| HS | hereditary spherocytosis | LSD | lysergic acid diethylamide |
| HSG | hysterosalpingography | LV | left ventricle, left ventricular |
| HSV | herpes simplex virus | LVH | left ventricular hypertrophy |
| HUS | hemolytic-uremic syndrome | Lytes | electrolytes |
| IABC | intra-aortic balloon counterpulsation | Mammo | mammography |
| | | MAO | monoamine oxidase (inhibitor) |
| ICA | internal carotid artery | MAP | mean arterial pressure |
| ICD | implantable cardiac defibrillator | MCA | middle cerebral artery |
| ICP | intracranial pressure | MCHC | mean corpuscular hemoglobin concentration |
| ICU | intensive care unit | | |
| ID/CC | identification and chief complaint | MCP | metacarpophalangeal (joint) |
| IDDM | insulin-dependent diabetes mellitus | MCV | mean corpuscular volume |
| | | MDMA | 3,4-methylene-dioxymethamphetamine ("ecstasy") |
| IE | infectious endocarditis | | |
| IFA | immunofluorescent antibody | MEN | multiple endocrine neoplasia |
| Ig | immunoglobulin | MGUS | monoclonal gammopathy of undetermined origin |
| IL | interleukin | | |
| IM | infectious mononucleosis, intramuscular | MHC | major histocompatibility complex |
| | | MI | myocardial infarction |
| INH | isoniazid | MIBG | metaiodobenzylguanidine |
| INR | International Normalized Ratio | MMR | measles, mumps, rubella (vaccine) |
| 123-ISS | iodine-123-labeled somatostatin | MPTP | 1-methyl-4-phenyl-tetrahydropyridine |
| IUD | intrauterine device | | |
| IUGR | intrauterine growth retardation | MR | magnetic resonance (imaging) |
| IV | intravenous | mRNA | messenger ribonucleic acid |
| IVC | inferior vena cava | MRSA | methicillin-resistant *Staphylococcus aureus* |
| IVIG | intravenous immunoglobulin | | |
| IVP | intravenous pyelography | MS | multiple sclerosis |
| JRA | juvenile rheumatoid arthritis | MTP | metatarsophalangeal (joint) |
| JVD | jugular venous distention | MuSK | muscle-specific kinase |
| JVP | jugular venous pressure | MVA | motor vehicle accident |
| KOH | potassium hydroxide | NADPH | reduced nicotinamide adenine dinucleotide phosphate |
| KS | Kaposis sarcoma | | |

| | |
|---|---|
| NAME | nevi, atrial myxoma, myxoid neurofibroma, ephilides (syndrome) |
| NG | nasogastric |
| NIDDM | non-insulin-dependent diabetes mellitus |
| NMDA | N-methyl-D-aspartate |
| NPO | nil per os (nothing by mouth) |
| NSAID | nonsteroidal anti-inflammatory drug |
| Nuc | nuclear medicine |
| OCD | obsessive-compulsive disorder |
| OCP | oral contraceptive pill |
| OCPD | obsessive-compulsive personality disorder |
| 17-OHP | 17-hydroxyprogesterone |
| OPC | organophosphate and carbamate |
| OS | opening snap |
| OTC | over the counter |
| PA | posteroanterior |
| 2-PAM | pralidoxime |
| P-ANCA | perinuclear antineutrophil cytoplasmic antibody |
| $PaO_2$ | partial pressure of oxygen |
| PAS | periodic acid Schiff |
| PBS | peripheral blood smear |
| $PCO_2$ | partial pressure of carbon dioxide |
| PCOD | polycystic ovary disease |
| PCP | phencyclidine |
| PCR | polymerase chain reaction |
| PCV | polycythemia vera |
| PDA | patent ductus arteriosus |
| PE | physical exam |
| PEEP | positive end-expiratory pressure |
| PET | positron emission tomography |
| PFTs | pulmonary function tests |
| PID | pelvic inflammatory disease |
| PIP | proximal interphalangeal (joint) |
| PKU | phenylketonuria |
| PMI | point of maximal impulse |
| PMN | polymorphonuclear (leukocyte) |
| PO | per os (by mouth) |
| $Po_2$ | partial pressure of oxygen |
| PPD | purified protein derivative |
| PROM | premature rupture of membranes |
| PRPP | phosphoribosyl pyrophosphate |
| PSA | prostate-specific antigen |
| PT | prothrombin time |
| PTE | pulmonary thromboembolism |
| PTH | parathyroid hormone |

| | |
|---|---|
| PTSD | post-traumatic stress disorder |
| PTT | partial thromboplastin time |
| RA | rheumatoid arthritis, right atrial |
| RBC | red blood cell |
| RDW | red-cell distribution width |
| REM | rapid eye movement |
| RF | rheumatoid factor |
| RhoGAM | Rh immune globulin |
| RNA | ribonucleic acid |
| RPR | rapid plasma reagin |
| RR | respiratory rate |
| RS | Reed–Sternberg (cell) |
| RSV | respiratory syncytial virus |
| RTA | renal tubular acidosis |
| RUQ | right upper quadrant |
| RV | residual volume, right ventricle, right ventricular |
| RVH | right ventricular hypertrophy |
| SA | sinoatrial |
| SAH | subarachnoid hemorrhage |
| $Sao_2$ | oxygen saturation in arterial blood |
| SBE | subacute bacterial endocarditis |
| SBFT | small bowel follow-through |
| SC | subcutaneous |
| SCC | squamous cell carcinoma |
| SIADH | syndrome of inappropriate secretion of antidiuretic hormone |
| SIDS | sudden infant death syndrome |
| SLE | systemic lupus erythematosus |
| SMA | smooth muscle antibody |
| SSPE | subacute sclerosing panencephalitis |
| SSRI | selective serotonin reuptake inhibitor |
| STD | sexually transmitted disease |
| SZPD | schizoid personality disorder |
| $T_3$ | triiodothyronine |
| $T_4$ | thyroxine |
| TAB | therapeutic abortion |
| TB | tuberculosis |
| TBSA | total body surface area |
| TCA | tricyclic antidepressant |
| TCD | transcranial Doppler |
| TD | tardive dyskinesia |
| TENS | transcutaneous electrical nerve stimulation |
| TFTs | thyroid function tests |
| THC | trans-tetrahydrocannabinol |
| TIA | transient ischemic attack |
| TIBC | total iron-binding capacity |

| | | | |
|---|---|---|---|
| TIPS | transjugular intrahepatic portosystemic shunt | URI | upper respiratory infection |
| | | US | ultrasound |
| TLC | total lung capacity | UTI | urinary tract infection |
| TMJ | temporomandibular joint (syndrome) | UV | ultraviolet |
| | | VCUG | voiding cystourethrogram |
| TMP-SMX | trimethoprim-sulfamethoxazole | VDRL | Venereal Disease Research Laboratory |
| TNF | tumor necrosis factor | | |
| TNM | tumor, node, metastasis (staging) | VF | ventricular fibrillation |
| ToRCH | *Toxoplasma,* rubella, CMV, herpes zoster | VIN | vulvar intraepithelial neoplasia |
| | | VLDL | very low density lipoprotein |
| tPA | tissue plasminogen activator | VMA | vanillylmandelic acid |
| TPO | thyroid peroxidase | V/Q | ventilation-perfusion (ratio) |
| TRAP | tartrate-resistant acid phosphatase | VS | vital signs |
| TRH | thyrotropin-releasing hormone | VSD | ventricular septal defect |
| TSH | thyroid-stimulating hormone | VT | ventricular tachycardia |
| TSS | toxic shock syndrome | vWF | von Willebrand factor |
| TSST | toxic shock syndrome toxin | VZIG | varicella-zoster immune globulin |
| TTP | thrombotic thrombocytopenic purpura | | |
| | | VZV | varicella-zoster virus |
| TUBD | transurethral balloon dilatation | WAGR | Wilms tumor, aniridia, ambiguous genitalia, mental retardation (syndrome) |
| TUIP | transurethral incision of the prostate | | |
| | | WBC | white blood cell |
| TURP | transurethral resection of the prostate | WG | Wegener granulomatosis |
| | | WPW | Wolff–Parkinson–White (syndrome) |
| UA | urinalysis | | |
| UGI | upper GI (series) | XR | x-ray |
| UMN | upper motor neuron | | |

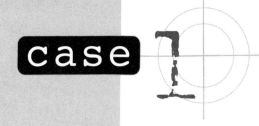

**ID/CC** A **25-year-old man** with a history of **IV drug abuse** presents to the ER complaining of **high fever with chills** and weakness.

**HPI** Over the past 2 weeks, the patient has had **intermittent spiking fevers** with **night sweats** and chills as well as associated **joint pain** (ARTHRALGIA). Recently, he has also become confused and disoriented.

**PE** VS: **fever** (39.5°C); tachycardia (HR 118); tachypnea (RR 25); normal BP. PE: pallor; 3/6 holosystolic **murmur** increasing with inspiration; tender, pulsatile liver edge; **Roth spots** observed on funduscopy; **Janeway lesions, Osler nodules,** splinter hemorrhages and petechiae on extremities.

**Labs** CBC: normocytic anemia; **leukocytosis** (16,300) with **left shift.** ESR and C-reactive protein elevated; **blood culture yields *Staphylococcus aureus.***

**Imaging** Echo (transesophageal): large, cauliflower-like **vegetation on the tricuspid valve; tricuspid regurgitation.**

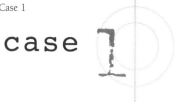

case 1

## Acute Bacterial Endocarditis

**Pathogenesis**

Acute bacterial endocarditis is characterized by the presence of **valvular vegetations** (composed of platelets and fibrin seeded by microorganisms carried in the blood) that tend to occur in areas of turbulent blood flow and carry a risk of embolism to a distant site. Classically, **subacute infectious endocarditis** is caused by organisms that rely on prior endocardial insults (*Streptococcus viridans*), and **acute infectious endocarditis** is caused by aggressive organisms such as *Staphylococcus aureus* that may infect normal native valves. Native valve endocarditis is also caused by *Streptococcus viridans*, group D streptococci, enterococci, and the so-called **HACEK organisms** (*Haemophilus, Actinobacillus, Cardiobacterium, Eikenella,* and *Kingella*).

**Epidemiology**

60% to 80% of patients have an underlying cardiac lesion (rheumatic heart disease, congenital heart lesions, mitral valve prolapse, aortic stenosis, or a prosthetic valve) that puts them at risk for endocarditis. The most commonly involved valves are, in order of frequency, the **mitral, aortic, tricuspid, and pulmonary valves.** Streptococci are the predominant organism in native valves of non–IV drug abusers. Among **IV drug abusers**, the **tricuspid valve** is classically involved, with *Staphylococcus aureus* as the most common pathogen.

**Management**

**IV antibiotics for 4 to 6 weeks** directed at the causative organism. Penicillin G and gentamicin are used for synergy to treat streptococci in native valve disease. Nafcillin and gentamicin can be used in IV drug users for methicillin-sensitive *Staphylococcus aureus*. In patients with prosthetic valves, vancomycin should be used for methicillin-resistant *Staphylococcus aureus*. **Valve replacement** is necessary in fungal or pseudomonal endocarditis, refractory congestive heart failure (due to valve incompetence), recurrent emboli, persistent bacteremia, complicated prosthetic valve involvement, and major myocardial involvement. After discharge, patients require lifelong **antibiotic prophylaxis** (amoxicillin or erythromycin) prior to dental work and other invasive procedures.

**Complications**

**Valvular destruction** may lead to pulmonary edema and congestive heart failure. **Septic emboli** may also occur, leading to distant infarction or infections. Deposition of immune complexes in the kidney may lead to **glomerulonephritis.** Local spread of infection may cause myocardial abscess, aortic root abscess, pericarditis, and myocardial infarction.

**Breakout Point**

- IV drug users at risk for tricuspid bacterial endocarditis
- Bicuspid aortic valve at risk for aortic bacterial endocarditis
- Janeway lesions, splinter hemorrhages, Roth spots, Osler nodes
- Antibiotic prophylaxis needed before dental work

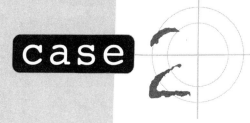

# case 2

**ID/CC**  A **50-year-old man** experiences an episode of **fainting** (SYNCOPE) while cleaning the house.

**HPI**  Within the past 6 months, he has felt increasing **fatigue, palpitations, chest pain,** and occasional **shortness of breath** (DYSPNEA).

**PE**  VS: tachycardia (HR 122); **wide pulse pressure** (BP 140/50). PE: tall (190 cm) with long, thin limbs and high-arched palate; dislocated lens (ECTOPIA LENTIS) in left eye (signs of Marfan syndrome); **bobbing movement of head** (DE MUSSET SIGN); crackles bilaterally at lung bases; **displaced PMI** (ventricular dilatation); $S_3$ over apex; **high-pitched, decrescendo, blowing diastolic murmur** loudest at left sternal border; systolic blushing and diastolic blanching with gentle pressure on nail bed (QUINCKE PULSE); **water-hammer pulse** (CORRIGAN SIGN).

**Labs**  ECG: sinus rhythm with increased QRS amplitude and left ventricular hypertrophy.

**Imaging**  CXR: LV enlargement with cardiac apex displaced downward and to left; enlarged ascending aorta. Echo: left ventricular hypertrophy; aortic root dilatation; flutter of anterior leaflet; early closure of mitral valve.

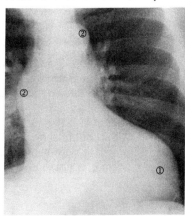

**Figure 2-1.**
CXR: LV enlargement *(1)* with cardiac apex displaced downward and to left; enlarged ascending aorta *(2)*.

# case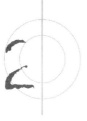

## Aortic Insufficiency

**Pathogenesis**

Aortic insufficiency (AORTIC REGURGITATION) may occur as a result of **rheumatic heart disease** (most common cause), **infective endocarditis**, Ehlers–Danlos syndrome (type IV), Marfan syndrome with either proximal root dilatation or aortic root dissection (secondary to cystic medial necrosis), idiopathic aortic root dissection, syphilitic aortitis, Takayasu arteritis, ankylosing spondylitis, Reiter syndrome, or congenital bicuspid valve. Aortic insufficiency leads to regurgitation of a fraction of the stroke volume back into the left ventricle during diastole, causing **increased LV filling pressure** and **end-diastolic volume**, which accounts for the **increased stroke volume and widened pulse pressure.** Ultimately, the increasing volume and filling pressure leads to congestive heart failure.

**Epidemiology**

**Aortic insufficiency is a common valvular lesion that** occurs more frequently in males. **However, in cases with concomitant mitral valve disease, females predominate.**

**Management**

Mild aortic insufficiency or asymptomatic severe aortic insufficiency, with normal heart size and no evidence of LV systolic dysfunction, requires only **bacterial endocarditis prophylaxis.** Symptomatic LV failure should be treated with **digitalis, diuretics, and vasodilators.** Patients with acute aortic insufficiency, medically refractory aortic insufficiency, increasing heart size, significant LV dysfunction, or decompensated congestive heart failure require **aortic valve replacement.** Beta-blockers can be used to slow the rate of aortic dilatation in Marfan syndrome.

**Complications**

Untreated, aortic insufficiency eventually leads to **congestive heart failure;** patients are also at risk for developing **arrhythmias** and **infective endocarditis.**

**Breakout Point**

- Presents as left ventricular failure or chest pain
- Wide pulse pressure
- Blowing diastolic murmur along left sternal border
- Enlarged, displaced LV

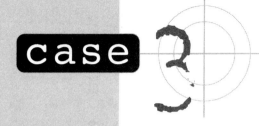

**ID/CC** A **60-year-old man** complains of left-sided **chest pain induced by exercise.**

**HPI** The patient states that he has experienced increasing **fatigue** and a decrease in his normal activity. He adds that he has **shortness of breath with exertion** and had one episode of **syncope** while playing football.

**PE** VS: tachycardia; narrow pulse pressure. PE: **delayed, slow-rising carotid upstroke (pulsus parvus et tardus);** forceful apical beat (**left ventricular hypertrophy**); **soft S$_2$** (secondary to diminished or absent aortic component); **harsh, late-peaking** (crescendo-decrescendo) **systolic ejection murmur** that is **loudest at right second intercostal space, radiating to carotids.**

**Labs** ECG: **left ventricular hypertrophy;** ST depression and T-wave inversion.

**Imaging** CXR: poststenotic dilatation of the ascending aorta; other findings include left ventricular hypertrophy with calcification of the aortic valve. Echo: **bicuspid aortic valve;** left ventricle wall thickening; decreased valvular area.

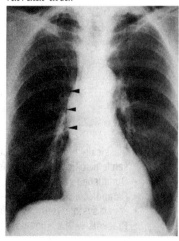

**Figure 3-1.** CXR. Poststenotic dilatation of the ascending aorta (*arrows*). Other findings include left ventricular hypertrophy with calcification of the aortic valve.

5

# case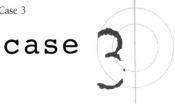

## Aortic Stenosis

**Pathogenesis**

Aortic stenosis may arise secondary to a **congenital bicuspid aortic valve** (60%), **rheumatic valvular disease** (10%), or idiopathic **senile calcific aortic stenosis** (common in the elderly). Obstruction to LV ejection leads to LV pressure overload and to a pressure gradient between the left ventricle and the aorta. In order to compensate for the increased wall stress, the left ventricle undergoes concentric hypertrophy, and **patients usually progress from angina to syncope to congestive heart failure.** Angina occurs as a result of increased oxygen demand coupled with decreased coronary artery perfusion; syncope occurs when the systemic vascular resistance drops during exercise while the cardiac output cannot increase sufficiently, leading to hypotension and poor cerebral perfusion.

**Epidemiology**

**Aortic stenosis is the** most common **cardiac valvular lesion; 80% of the symptomatic adults are male.**

**Management**

**Aortic valve replacement** for **symptomatic** patients and for **asymptomatic** patients with very severe left ventricular hypertrophy, a significantly reduced valve area ($\leq 0.7$ cm$^2$), and high pressure gradients. **Pharmacologic therapy** has a limited role. Digitalis and salt restriction may be used for palliation of congestive heart failure symptoms. Use diuretics cautiously and avoid vasodilators (versus aortic insufficiency). Patients should **avoid strenuous activity** and should receive **antibiotic prophylaxis** for all invasive medical and dental procedures.

**Complications**

Congestive heart failure may result. Sudden cardiac death may occur, presumably due to ventricular arrhythmias. Supraventricular arrhythmias, systemic emboli, and infective endocarditis may occur. Patients also have increased risk of arteriovenous malformations.

**Breakout Point**

- Classically in congenital bicuspid aortic valve or senile calcific aortic stenosis
- Diminished carotid pulses
- Paradoxically split S2
- Harsh systolic murmur radiating to the neck
- Presents with syncope, angina, and dyspnea

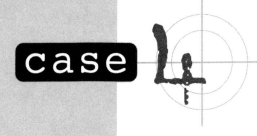

**case** 4

**ID/CC**  A **39-year-old woman** complains of recent-onset shortness of breath (DYSPNEA), **fatigue**, and **decreased exercise tolerance.**

**HPI**  She states that the shortness of breath is **exacerbated when she stands and is relieved when she lies down.** She also states that she has developed **palpitations, malaise,** and **joint pains.** She has lost approximately 30 pounds in the past year.

**PE**  VS: **low-grade fever;** tachycardia; postural hypotension. PE: cachexia; clubbing; pallor; increased JVP; loud $S_1$; **low-pitched sound in early diastole** ("TUMOR PLOP" from myxoma stopping when it strikes the ventricular wall); Raynaud phenomenon can be seen.

**Labs**  CBC: anemia (hemolytic); leukocytosis; thrombocytopenia. **ESR elevated;** hypergammaglobulinemia. ECG: sinus tachycardia.

**Imaging**  CXR: enlarged left atrium, pulmonary vascular redistribution, and RV enlargement. Echo: single, mobile, **intracavitary,** pedunculated **mass in left atrium.**

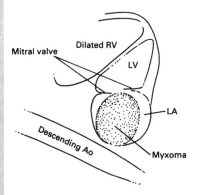

**Figure 4-1.** Echo (schematic). Single, mobile, **intracavitary,** pedunculated **mass in left atrium.**

# case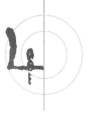

## Atrial Myxoma

**Pathogenesis**

Myxomas are true neoplasms that arise most commonly from the **left atrial septum** near the fossa ovalis; they are generally solitary, pedunculated, and 4 to 8 cm in diameter. These tumors frequently prolapse through the atrioventricular valve, yielding symptoms similar to **valvular stenosis**. However, they may also cause valvular trauma, leading to symptoms of **regurgitation**. In a small percentage of cases, the tumors are transmitted in an **autosomal-dominant** fashion. They may also arise as part of the NAME (NEVI, ATRIAL MYXOMA, MYXOID NEUROFIBROMA, EPHELIDES) or LAMB (LENTIGINES, ATRIAL MYXOMA, BLUE NEVI) syndromes.

**Epidemiology**

Although the majority of tumors involving the heart are metastatic in origin, myxomas are the **most common primary cardiac tumor**. There is a female predominance, with most tumors presenting between the third and sixth decades of life, or earlier when familial or associated with a syndrome.

**Management**

**Surgical excision;** screen first-degree relatives in young patients and those with multiple tumors.

**Complications**

Congestive heart failure, sudden death, arrhythmias, infection, and embolization.

**Breakout Point**

- Most common primary cardiac tumor in adults
- More common in left atrium (rather than right atrium)
- "Ball-valve" effect that can obstruct blood flow

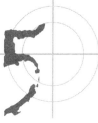

# case 5

**ID/CC** A **40-year-old woman** complains of **progressive shortness of breath** (SOB) for 2 weeks.

**HPI** She has a history of **melanoma** (diagnosed 10 years ago, s/p surgical resection) and hypertension. Initially, her SOB was on exertion, but over the past 2 days it has been present even at rest. She denies fever, chills, orthopnea, or paroxysmal nocturnal dyspnea.

**PE** VS: **tachycardia** (HR 130), **tachypnea** (RR 30). PE: **positive jugular venous distension;** regular rate and rhythm; **distant heart sounds; pulsus paradoxus;** bilateral inspiratory crackles and 2+ lower-extremity edema.

**Labs** CBC: normocytic anemia; lytes: hyponatremia; mild creatinine elevation. Normal cardiac enzymes. UA: normal.

**Imaging** ECG: regular rhythm, sinus tachycardia, low-voltage QRS, electrical alternans.

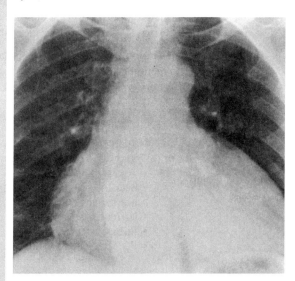

**Figure 5-1.** Globular enlargement of the cardiac silhouette reflects a pericardial effusion.

case 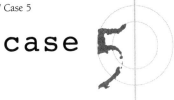 5

## Cardiac Tamponade

**Pathogenesis**

Cardiac tamponade is a clinical syndrome that results from fluid filling of the pericardial sac impairing ventricular filling and, therefore, cardiac output. Signs and symptoms include the **Beck triad (jugular venous distention, hypotension, and muffled heart sounds), dyspnea, tachycardia** (to compensate for the low stroke volume), and **pulsus paradoxus** (inspiratory drop of systolic blood pressure of more than 10 mm Hg). It may present in an acute manner due to rapid accumulation of fluid as in trauma, ventricular wall rupture (iatrogenic or post-MI), and dissecting aortic aneurysm. It may also be subacute or chronic as with infectious pericarditis, neoplasms (breast, lung, melanoma, Hodgkin disease), autoimmune disease, and metabolic derangements (uremia, hypothyroidism). Chest x-ray can show cardiomegaly with a globular shape. ECG shows sinus tachycardia, low voltage, and beat-to-beat alternation in the amplitude of QRS complex (electrical alternans).

**Management**

**Hemodynamic instability is an indication for urgent pericardiocentesis.** The use of inotropes is controversial, but fluid resuscitation is recommended. Management should be directed to evaluate the etiology of pericardial effusion.

**Complications**

**Cardiogenic shock** causing hypoperfusion to vital organs leading to multiorgan failure.

**Breakout Point**

- Beck triad: jugular venous distension, muffled heart sounds, hypotension
- Narrow pulse pressure
- Pulsus paradoxus
- Pericardial friction rub

# case 6

**ID/CC** A 79-year-old **woman** complains of **severe shortness of breath** (DYSPNEA) at rest.

**HPI** The patient states that she suffered a **myocardial infarct** 1 year ago. Since then she **needs three pillows to sleep** (ORTHOPNEA) and sometimes **wakes up at night coughing,** with shortness of breath (PAROXYSMAL NOCTURNAL DYSPNEA). Additionally, she notes a loss of appetite (ANOREXIA).

**PE** VS: **tachycardia** (HR 130); **tachypnea** (RR 34); **normal BP.** PE: in acute distress; diaphoretic; cyanotic; **JVD; bilateral rales;** PMI displaced downward and to left; $S_3$ and $S_4$ heard; **tender hepatomegaly; pedal edema.**

**Labs** LFTs: mildly elevated hepatic enzymes (due to hepatic congestion). ECG: Q-waves in $V_1$ through $V_4$ (old anterior wall myocardial infarct); ST elevation in leads $V_5$ and $V_6$ (acute lateral wall ischemia).

**Imaging** CXR: cardiomegaly; prominent pulmonary vasculature; interstitial pulmonary edema. Echo: akinetic anterior wall; LV ejection fraction 30%.

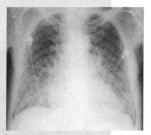

**Figure 6-1.** CXR. Cardiomegaly; prominent pulmonary vasculature; interstitial pulmonary edema.

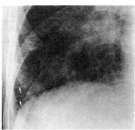

**Figure 6-2.** CXR. **Kerley B** lines (*arrows*) are found in the peripheral lung bases and are manifestations of interstitial pulmonary edema.

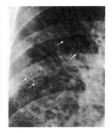

**Figure 6-3.** CXR. Kerley A lines (*arrows*) are seen more toward the lung apices.

case 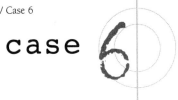 6

## Congestive Heart Failure

**Pathogenesis**

Congestive heart failure (CHF) represents a syndrome characterized by inability of the heart to provide adequate forward flow to meet the metabolic demands of the body's tissues **(defined as systolic heart failure)**, or the inability to meet metabolic demands at high filling pressure **(diastolic heart failure)**. Systolic dysfunction arises in conditions that lead to decreased contractility (myocardial infarct, toxic cardiomyopathy) or increased afterload (severe chronic hypertension, dilated cardiomyopathy, and aortic stenosis). Conversely, diastolic dysfunction arises as a result of impaired active relaxation (myocardial ischemia, ventricular hypertrophy) or passive relaxation (amyloidosis, constrictive pericarditis).

**Epidemiology**

>750,000 individuals per year die from heart disease in the United States. **The vast majority of these deaths are attributable to ischemic heart disease, hypertensive heart disease and cor pulmonale, valvular disease, and congenital disease.** Congestive heart failure is the final common pathway of these conditions.

**Management**

In the absence of pure diastolic dysfunction, therapy should be directed at **increasing contractility** with cardiac glycosides such as digitalis. **Reduction of preload and afterload** can be achieved through use of ACE inhibitors, beta-blockers, and diuretics. Diuretics are the most effective means of providing symptomatic relief, and adding spironolactone to furosemide in patients with severe congestive heart failure has been found to provide added benefit. When pulmonary edema is present, oxygen, diuretics, morphine, and vasodilators are frequently indicated. Therapy should be directed toward treating the underlying etiology of congestive heart failure. A low-salt diet should be encouraged.

**Complications**

Hypoxic encephalopathy, prerenal azotemia, and death.

**Breakout Point**

- Jugular venous distension
- S3 and S4
- Bibasilar crackles
- Most common cause of right heart failure is left heart failure

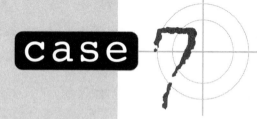

**ID/CC**    A **60-year-old man** presents with progressive, **severe shortness of breath** (DYSPNEA) and **cough.**

**HPI**    The patient is a **chronic smoker** and has been receiving treatment for **COPD.** He reports **swollen feet** and an increase in **abdominal girth.**

**PE**    VS: tachycardia (HR 120); tachypnea (RR 30); weight gain (due to fluid retention); hypoxia ($SaO_2$ 88% on room air). PE: moderate **respiratory distress;** central cyanosis present; **JVP elevated;** bilateral pitting **pedal edema; bilateral rhonchi and crepitations,** the character of which changes with coughing; palpable left parasternal heave; loud $P_2$ and **RV $S_3$;** ascites and mildly **tender hepatomegaly.**

**Labs**    ABGs: **hypoxia and respiratory alkalosis.** CBC: elevated hematocrit (55%). ECG: right axis deviation; **P pulmonale;** right ventricular hypertrophy.

**Imaging**    CXR: enlargement of the hilar vasculature; prominence of the main pulmonary artery; relative cardiomegaly given the degree of hyperinflation. Echo: **right ventricular dilatation.** US, abdomen: **congestive hepatomegaly** and ascites.

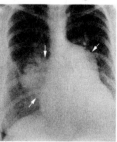

**Figure 7-1.** CXR. Enlargement of the hilar vasculature (*arrows on left*); prominence of the main pulmonary artery (*arrow on right*); relative cardiomegaly given the degree of hyperinflation.

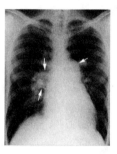

**Figure 7-2.** CXR. Another case, again showing a massive main pulmonary artery and cardiomegaly.

13

# case 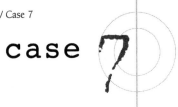 7

## Cor Pulmonale

**Pathogenesis** — Cor pulmonale is defined as **intrinsic disease of the lungs, thorax, or pulmonary circulation that induces right ventricular changes.** Pulmonary hypertension eventually increases right ventricular afterload and ultimately results in right ventricular failure. Although the **most common cause is COPD,** other causes include primary pulmonary hypertension, chronic bronchitis, recurrent pulmonary embolism, sickle-cell anemia, interstitial lung disease, bronchiectasis, chronic bronchial asthma, cystic fibrosis, myasthenia gravis, ankylosing spondylitis, and vasculitis.

**Epidemiology** — Prevalence is determined by the underlying cause of cor pulmonale.

**Management** — **Correct alveolar hypoxia** by judiciously **increasing the inspired $O_2$ concentration** (ventilation is in part driven by hypoxia in these patients) and improving alveolar ventilation by relieving the airway obstruction **(bronchodilators and steroids). Diuretics** relieve the edema. **Restrict sodium intake; quit smoking;** avoid alcohol and sedatives.

**Complications** — Supraventricular or ventricular arrhythmias and biventricular cardiac failure are common complications.

**Breakout Point**

- Most common cause in the United States—COPD
- Intrinsic lung disease that causes right heart failure

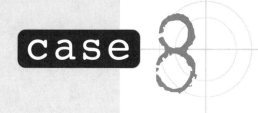

| | |
|---|---|
| **ID/CC** | A **50-year-old man** experiences progressive **shortness of breath** and pronounced intolerance of physical activity. |
| **HPI** | He also complains of cough and swelling of his ankles. He is in his seventh month of chemotherapy (including **daunorubicin**) for non-Hodgkin lymphoma. |
| **PE** | VS: tachycardia; mild hypotension (BP 100/60); tachypnea. PE: respiratory distress; faint rales heard bilaterally; **elevated JVP**; $S_3$ gallop rhythm; **holosystolic murmur** in mitral and tricuspid areas; **2+ pitting edema** in lower extremities. |
| **Labs** | CBC: normal. **Increased BUN and creatinine;** BUN/creatinine ratio >20 (sign of prerenal azotemia). Lytes: **hyponatremia.** ECG: sinus tachycardia. |
| **Imaging** | CXR: sinus tachycardia with cardiomegaly. |

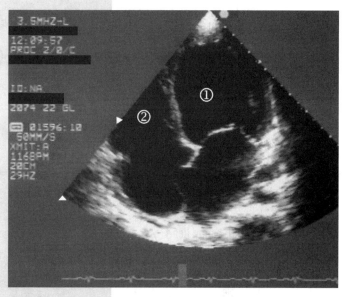

**Figure 8-1.** Echo. LV (*1*) and RV (*2*) dilatation and systolic dysfunction (reduced EF).

# case 8

## Dilated Cardiomyopathy

**Pathogenesis**

Most cases of dilated cardiomyopathy are **idiopathic**; other causes include **long-standing hypertension, alcohol abuse, postpartum, beriberi, coxsackievirus** infection, and **cocaine abuse**. In this case, heart failure was most likely secondary to chemotherapy with **daunorubicin**. Dilated cardiomyopathy usually presents clinically as congestive heart failure secondary to diminished LV function and decreased CO.

**Epidemiology**

Most cases are sporadic. 20% of patients demonstrate familial forms with various modes of genetic transmission.

**Management**

Diuretics, ACE inhibitors, vasodilators (nitrates), and digitalis are used to treat congestive heart failure symptoms. With diminished left ventricular function, oral anticoagulation may be considered due to the high risk of atrial and ventricular arrhythmia and thromboembolization. **Vaccination** with influenza and pneumococcal vaccines is recommended. **Cardiac transplantation** may be considered in severe cases which are irreversible. In reversible causes of dilated cardiomyopathy (alcohol abuse, selenium deficiency, hypophosphatemia, hypocalcemia, thyroid disease, cocaine use, and chronic uncontrolled tachycardia), the underlying etiology should be addressed.

**Complications**

Complications include deterioration of ventricular function followed by death (due to **arrhythmias** or **intractable congestive heart failure**). Systemic and pulmonary thromboembolic complications may also occur.

**Breakout Point**

- Big, baggy heart
- Presents as congestive heart failure (jugular venous distension, S3 and S4, dependent edema)
- Alcoholic dilated cardiomyopathy can be reversible

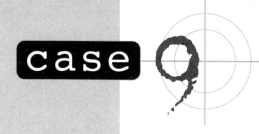

**case 9**

| | |
|---|---|
| **ID/CC** | A **62-year-old man** with a history of **diabetes mellitus type 2** and **hypertension** presents for a routine visit to his primary care physician. |
| **HPI** | He has been feeling well with no complaints. He denies headaches, visual changes, chest pain, back pain, or abdominal pain. |
| **PE** | VS: hypertensive (BP **230/120**), unchanged supine or standing. VS: no evidence of papilledema or retinal hemorrhages, lungs clear, neurologic exam normal. |
| **Labs** | CBC/Lytes: normal. Urine toxin screen: negative for cocaine and amphetamines. |
| **Imaging** | ECG: **left ventricular hypertrophy.** CT head: normal. |

# case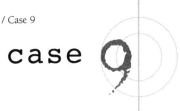

## Hypertensive Urgency

**Pathogenesis**

Hypertensive urgency is described as **elevated blood pressure without evidence of end-organ damage.** Classically, systolic pressure is >220 mm Hg and diastolic pressure is >120 mm Hg, but end-organ damage is the true distinguishing factor between hypertensive urgency and hypertensive emergency, regardless of specific measurements of blood pressure. Hypertensive urgency warrants a **controlled blood pressure reduction.**

**Epidemiology**

Hypertensive urgency occurs in approximately 1% of hypertensive patients.

**Management**

The initial goal of therapy in hypertensive urgency is to **achieve a diastolic BP of 100 to 110 mm Hg** or a 25% reduction of the mean arterial pressure **within several hours.** Excessive or rapid decreases in BP should be avoided to minimize the risk of cerebral hypoperfusion or coronary insufficiency. Normal blood pressure can be attained gradually over several days as tolerated by the individual patient. Once blood pressure has been reduced via oral medications, institution of additional antihypertensive medications and/or their adjustments can be done as an outpatient with gradual titration.

**Breakout Point**

- Either asymptomatic or no new end-organ damage
- Hypertension should be decreased in a controlled way, not ourly rapidly for risk of end-organ ischemia

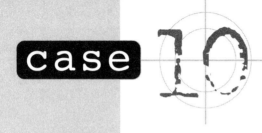

case 10

**ID/CC**   A **20-year-old man** is brought to the ER after **collapsing** during a tennis match.

**HPI**   He states that his father was forced to quit his college basketball team after episodes of syncope.

**PE**   VS: mild hypertension (BP 140/90); **tachycardia** (HR 132); tachypnea. PE: brisk carotid upstroke with palpable double impulse; **double apical cardiac impulse,** prominent $S_4$, and **coarse systolic outflow murmur** localized along left sternal border and accentuated by the Valsalva maneuver.

**Labs**   ECG: left axis deviation (due to left ventricular hypertrophy), septal Q-wave, and right bundle branch block. Muscle biopsy reveals myocardial disarray.

**Imaging**   CXR: evidence of left atrial and ventricular enlargement. Echo: increased thickness of the ventricular septum, enhanced contractility, and signs of dynamic obstruction.

case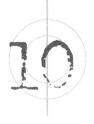

## Hypertrophic Obstructive Cardiomyopathy

**Pathogenesis**

Hypertrophic obstructive cardiomyopathy is characterized by the presence of **heterogenous left ventricular hypertrophy** (usually with preferential left ventricular septal hypertrophy) in association with a **dynamic left ventricular outflow tract pressure gradient** (due to midsystolic apposition of the anterior mitral valve leaflet against the hypertrophic septum, resulting in a subaortic narrowing). **Obstruction is worsened by decreased left ventricular filling (Valsalva maneuver, vasodilators) or by increased myocardial contractility (digoxin).** Decreased compliance of the hypertrophic muscle results in elevated diastolic filling pressures, leading to diastolic dysfunction.

**Epidemiology**

A genetic component (with **autosomal-dominant** inheritance) has been observed in about half of all cases. Hypertrophic obstructive cardiomyopathy is the most common cause of sudden death in young athletes.

**Management**

Key management components include avoidance of strenuous physical activity; beta-blockers (to reduce heart rate and cardiac contractility); calcium-channel blockers, particularly verapamil and diltiazem (to augment diastolic ventricular filling); and surgery (septal myomectomy) for cases that are unresponsive to medical therapy.

**Complications**

Atrial fibrillation, systemic embolization, sudden death, and infective endocarditis.

**Breakout Point**

- Presents as dyspnea, chest pain, syncope
- Outflow tract obstruction
- Systolic ejection murmur that increases with Valsalva maneuver
- Family history of syncope or sudden death

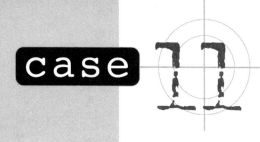

# case 11

**ID/CC**  A **65-year-old man** with end-stage prostate cancer develops **dyspnea on exertion**, fever, and fatigue.

**HPI**  He has a 25-pack-year smoking history. He was diagnosed with **prostate cancer** at age 62. Aggressive therapy was abandoned 2 months ago. He reports multiple transient neurologic symptoms.

**PE**  VS: **wide pulse pressure** (BP 146/52); **tachycardia** (HR 112); bounding pulses; tachypnea. PE: **diastolic murmur** localized at right sternal border; full hard pulse followed by sudden collapse (CORRIGAN PULSE); rhythmic nodding of head synchronous with heartbeat (DE MUSSET SIGN); loud "pistol shot" heard on auscultation over femoral arteries (TRAUBE SIGN) (signs of aortic insufficiency).

**Labs**  CBC/Lytes: normal. **Blood cultures negative.**

**Imaging**  None.

# case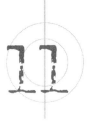

## Marantic Endocarditis

**Pathogenesis**

Marantic endocarditis is characteristically associated with terminal illnesses such as **cancer** (commonly adenocarcinomas and promyelocytic leukemia). Pathologically, cardiac valves reveal the presence of small, **sterile fibrin deposits** (vegetations) distributed along the lines of closure of the leaflets or cusps.

**Management**

Aortic valve replacement is not indicated because the patient has end-stage cancer. Therapy should be directed toward minimization of symptoms. Prevention involves treatment of underlying cause—in this case, prostate cancer.

**Complications**

Sequelae of valvular heart disease, including congestive heart failure, arterial embolization, and resultant tissue infarction.

**Breakout Point**

- Sterile vegetations that do not contain bacteria
- Associated with cancer or sepsis

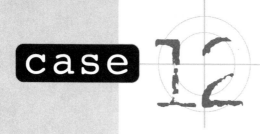

**ID/CC** A **56-year-old man** who suffered an acute non–Q-wave anterolateral MI is found to have a new murmur during his third day post–MI.

**HPI** He has a history of coronary artery disease. He was admitted for severe precordial chest pain that lasted for a few hours. On day 3 he began to complain of increasing dyspnea and fatigue.

**PE** PE: in mild distress; brisk carotid upstroke; diffuse bibasilar rales; prominent $S_3$; **3/6 pansystolic murmur best heard at the apex with radiation to the axilla;** hyperdynamic LV impulse; distal pulses intact; no peripheral edema.

**Labs** CBC/Lytes: normal. CPK mildly elevated; CK-MB fraction elevated; mildly elevated troponin I; Swan–Ganz catheter was placed, demonstrating **no step-up in blood oxygen saturation** from right atrium to pulmonary artery; **giant V-waves** (corresponding to ventricular systole) noted on pressure tracings. ECG: left atrial enlargement.

**Imaging** Echo: flail mitral leaflet with papillary muscle rupture.

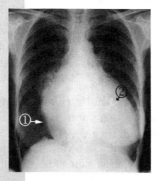

**Figure 12-1.** CXR. A case showing massive enlargement of the right heart border (*1*), prominence of the main pulmonary artery, and calcification of the mitral valve (*2*).

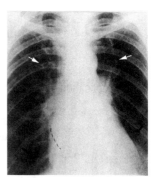

**Figure 12-2.** CXR. A different case showing "cephalization" (upper zone vessels are larger than equivalent vessels in the lower lung zones) (*arrows*).

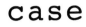 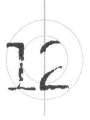

## Mitral Insufficiency

Pathogenesis
: Mitral valve insufficiency is most commonly secondary to myxomatous degeneration (**mitral valve prolapse**), valve perforation (**infective endocarditis**), subvalvular dysfunction (**papillary muscle dysfunction or ruptured chordae tendineae due to acute MI**), **rheumatic heart disease** (was once the most common cause), or rarely, cardiac tumors (left atrial myxoma).

Management
: Proper management relies on **accurate identification of the underlying cause.** Doppler studies provide both qualitative and semiquantitative estimates of mitral regurgitation severity. Cardiac catheterization provides accurate assessment of regurgitation, LV function, and pulmonary artery pressures. Coronary angiography defines underlying coronary disease present prior to valvular repair. Administration of nitroprusside or intra-aortic balloon counterpulsation (IABC) may reduce regurgitation or shunt, but **emergent surgical repair** is often indicated in cases of acute mitral regurgitation due to MI, endocarditis, or ruptured chordae tendineae. Chronic mitral insufficiency may remain asymptomatic for years and may require surgical repair only upon progressive deterioration of LV function or when disease becomes activity-limiting.

Complications
: Mitral insufficiency is a risk factor for severe pulmonary edema, cardiogenic shock, atrial fibrillation, and infective endocarditis. Ventricular tachycardias and sudden death are rare.

Breakout Point
: 
- Holosystolic murmur heard best at the apex
- Radiates to the axilla
- May be asymptomatic for many years
- Second most common valvular disease (after aortic stenosis)

# case 13

**ID/CC** A **35-year-old woman** presents with **hemoptysis**, progressively increasing **exertional dyspnea**, and **paroxysmal nocturnal dyspnea**.

**HPI** She reports a childhood history of fever accompanied by joint pain and skin rash **(acute rheumatic fever)**; since that time she has been diagnosed with a valvular heart disease and has been receiving penicillin injections every 3 weeks.

**PE** VS: low-volume pulse. PE: mild peripheral cyanosis (due to reduced cardiac output); left parasternal heave; loud $S_1$ and $P_2$; **"rumbling" mid-diastolic murmur** with presystolic accentuation heard at apex; **opening snap** heard at apex.

**Labs** ECG: P mitrale; RVH.

**Imaging** CXR: left atrial enlargement; pulmonary venous congestion. Barium swallow: narrowing of the esophagus by enlarged left atrium. Echo: fusion of commissures causes the posterior leaflet to move anteriorly with the anterior leaflet rather than in its usual posterior direction during diastole.

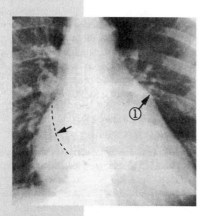

**Figure 13-1.** CXR. Left atrial enlargement (*1 and arrows*); pulmonary venous congestion.

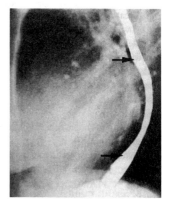

**Figure 13-2.** Barium swallow. Narrowing of the esophagus (*arrows*) by enlarged left atrium.

# case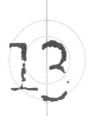

## Mitral Stenosis

**Pathogenesis**

Mitral stenosis is generally **rheumatic in origin;** rarely it may be congenital (e.g., ASD with acquired mitral stenosis—Lutembacher syndrome). Mitral stenosis and mitral insufficiency often coexist.

**Epidemiology**

Two-thirds of all patients with mitral stenosis are females. Pure or predominant mitral stenosis occurs in approximately 40% of all patients with rheumatic heart disease. The occurrence of mitral stenosis is decreasing in developed countries owing to the declining incidence of rheumatic fever.

**Management**

**Because mitral stenosis is usually asymptomatic for many years, no treatment may be required for a long time.** Pregnancy (increased cardiac output and transmural pressure gradient) or atrial fibrillation may precipitate severe symptoms. Patients with **atrial fibrillation** should be converted to and maintained in sinus rhythm with **digoxin or anti-arrhythmics** and should be given **warfarin** anticoagulation to prevent embolic events. Most patients do not require **surgical therapy** until they develop (1) recalcitrant pulmonary edema, (2) activity-limiting dyspnea and pulmonary edema, (3) pulmonary hypertension with RVH or hemoptysis, (4) activity limitation despite ventricular rate control and medical therapy, or (5) recurrent systemic emboli despite anticoagulation. **Open mitral valve commissurotomy** is effective in most patients in the absence of substantial regurgitation. **Balloon valvuloplasty** is an increasingly common procedure for patients without regurgitation. **Valve replacement** is the definitive treatment; it is performed for critical mitral stenosis, mitral incompetence, calcified valves, left atrial thrombus, and floppy valves. All patients with rheumatic heart disease should receive **prophylactic antibiotics** prior to dental, surgical, and urologic procedures to prevent endocarditis. Women with known disease should be counseled regarding the risks associated with pregnancy.

**Complications**

Patients may develop pulmonary hypertension, right heart failure, atrial fibrillation, systemic and cerebral embolization, and bacterial endocarditis.

**Breakout Point**

- Diastolic rumbling murmur heard best at the apex
- Opening snap
- Presents as orthopnea, paroxysmal nocturnal dyspnea
- Often precipitated by atrial fibrillation or pregnancy

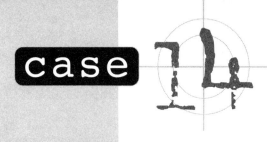

**ID/CC** A **67-year-old man** complains of chest pain over the last 30 minutes.

**HPI** He describes a severe, **substernal pressure across his chest** radiating to the shoulders. The pain awoke him from sleep. He also complains of nausea, fatigue, and perspiration.

**PE** VS: normal. PE: bibasilar crackles in lungs; S4 but no murmurs or rubs; weak dorsalis pedis, posterior tibialis pulses bilaterally.

**Labs** Cardiac biomarkers (CK, CK-MB, troponin I): elevated. CBC: WBC mildly elevated.

**Imaging** CXR: mild interstitial thickening. No mediastinal widening. ECG: acute ST-elevation with involvement of proximal left anterior descending artery.

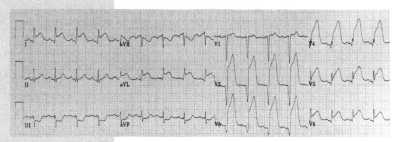

**Figure 14-1.** ST-segment elevation in leads I, aVL, V1–V6 as well as ST-segment depression in III and aVF, suggests proximal left anterior descending artery occlusion.

case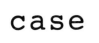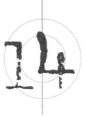

## Myocardial Infarction

**Pathogenesis**

Myocardial infarctions result from the disruption of athero-sclerotic plaques in coronary arteries. Exposure of plaque contents to circulating blood triggers platelet adhesion, activation, and aggregation, and the formation of a platelet plug. Plaque rupture also triggers the coagulation cascade and formation of a fibrin clot. Coronary artery occlusion by a **thrombus** composed of platelets, fibrin, and red blood cells causes myocardial necrosis. Necrosis involving the entire thickness of the myocardium (**transmural** injury) usually causes ST-segment elevations. Restricted **subendocardial** injury can also result from coronary artery occlusion and is typically associated with ST-segment depression. Q-waves may develop in either type of infarction.

**Management**

MI management revolves around the rapid restoration of blood supply to the injured myocardium through **fibrinolytic therapy** and/or **percutaneous angioplasty and/or stenting.** Antiplatelet agents such as **aspirin, beta-blockers, clopidogrel, heparin,** and **GP IIb/IIIa inhibitors** help limit the formation of a platelet plug around an unstable plaque. Antithrombin agents, such as heparin, also help establish and maintain patency in the affected artery. Beta-blockers help limit infarct size but are avoided in infarcts complicated by cardiogenic shock. Nitrates and morphine are useful analgesics but their use requires a clinical assessment of hemodynamics and mental status.

**Complications**

Myocardial wall rupture, papillary muscle rupture, and post-MI arrhythmias can result.

**Breakout Point**

- Oxygen, aspirin, heparin, clopidogral, beta-blockers are the cornerstone of treatment
- CK-MB increases at 6 hours, peaks at 24 hours, returns to normal in 3 to 4 days
- Troponin increases at 6 hours, peaks at 48 hours, returns to normal in 7 to 10 days
- Inferior leads: II, III, AVF; lateral leads: I, AVL, V5-V6; anteroseptal leads: V1-V3

# case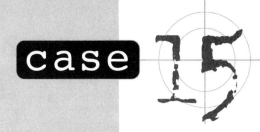

| | |
|---|---|
| ID/CC | A **25-year-old woman** presents with episodic attacks of **dizziness, shortness of breath,** and **palpitations.** |
| HPI | She is taking verapamil daily for a heart condition. |
| PE | VS: tachycardia (HR 150); hypotension (BP 90/50). PE: JVP normal; normal $S_1$ and $S_2$; remainder of systemic exam normal. |
| Labs | ECG: Rate 150 bpm **regular narrow QRS complexes without preceding P-waves.** |
| Imaging | CXR: normal. |

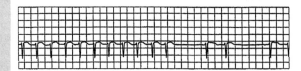

**Figure 15-1.** Narrow QRS complexes without preceding P-waves that terminates and converts to sinus rhythm.

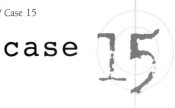

# case

## Paroxysmal Supraventricular Tachycardia

**Pathogenesis**

Most cases of paroxysmal supraventricular tachycardia are caused by **reentry** at one of three sites: (1) in the AV node in about 40% to 50% of cases; (2) over a concealed, extranodal accessory bypass tract in 30% to 40% of cases; or (3) in the sinus node or atria in 5% to 10% of cases.

**Epidemiology**

The condition is **very common** and is often experienced by people with **structurally normal hearts.** It is frequently seen in preexcitation syndromes and in association with certain congenital abnormalities, such as ASD and Ebstein anomaly. It also occurs in patients with rheumatic, atherosclerotic, hypertensive, or thyrotoxic heart disease; may occur following MI; and may be **precipitated by stress, tobacco, caffeine, or alcohol.**

**Management**

Treatment is aimed at blocking AV node conduction, including the use of **vagal maneuvers** for acute attacks (e.g., carotid sinus massage). Vagal maneuvers are contraindicated in the presence of carotid bruits or a history of transient cerebral ischemic attacks. If unsuccessful, attempt pharmacologic therapy. **IV adenosine** is currently the drug of choice because of its short half-life. **IV verapamil** is also considered a first-line agent. Beta-blockers are second-line agents and should not be used concurrently with calcium-channel blockers (may cause sinus arrest or severe hypotension). **Digoxin** should not be used acutely because of its prolonged onset of action. **Cardioversion is the initial treatment of choice when there is marked hypotension,** severe angina, or cardiovascular collapse, or when pharmacologic measures fail; do not use when digitalis toxicity is suspected. **Radiofrequency catheter ablation** is now the treatment of choice for long-term suppression in patients with symptomatic supraventricular tachycardias associated with manifest accessory atrioventricular pathways (e.g., Wolff–Parkinson–White syndrome), concealed accessory atrioventricular pathways, and AV nodal reentry. Pharmacologic therapies for the chronic suppression of paroxysmal supraventricular tachycardia include calcium-channel blockers, beta-blockers, and digoxin.

**Complications**

LV failure may result from coexistent structural heart disease. Complications also rarely include ventricular arrhythmias, myocardial infarct, congestive heart failure, syncope, and sudden death.

**Breakout Point**

- Very common
- Presents as palpitations and dizziness
- Structurally normal heart caused by re-entry in the AV node, accessory by pass tract, or in the sinus node or atria

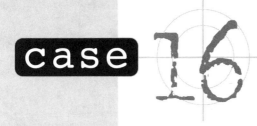

**case 16**

| | |
|---|---|
| ID/CC | A **27-year-old man** presents with **chest pain** and low-grade **fever** of 1 week's duration. |
| HPI | His pain is described as **retrosternal and radiates to his back, worsens with deep inspiration,** and is **relieved when he sits up and leans forward.** |
| PE | VS: normal. PE: tachycardia with regular rhythm; triphasic, **high-pitched scratching sound heard over left lower sternal border** (PERICARDIAL FRICTION RUB). |
| Labs | ECG: **PR-segment depression and diffuse ST-segment elevation** with an upright T-wave; later stages show inverted T-waves without Q-waves. |
| Imaging | Echo: good cardiac function with small pericardial effusion. CXR: normal. |

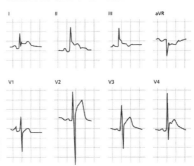

**Figure 16-1. ECG. PR-segment depression and diffuse ST-segment elevation** with an upright T-wave; later stages show inverted T-waves without Q-waves.

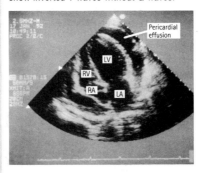

**Figure 16-2.** Echo. Good cardiac function with small pericardial effusion.

31

# case 16

## Pericarditis

### Pathogenesis

**Viral infections** (coxsackie B, echovirus, HIV) are the most common cause of acute pericarditis. Other causes include bacterial infections (*Pneumococcus, Staphylococcus, Meningococcus, Mycobacterium tuberculosis,* and *Haemophilus influenzae*), fungal infections (*Histoplasma capsulatum*), uremia, hypothyroidism, drug-induced pericarditis (procainamide and minoxidil), **radiation-induced** pericardial effusion (common in patients who have received large doses of radiation to the mediastinum), **neoplasms** (most often with breast or lung cancer), postcardiac surgery or postcardiotomy syndrome, **post-MI immune-mediated pericarditis** (DRESSLER SYNDROME), and **autoimmune disorders** (SLE, RA).

### Epidemiology

The incidence of tuberculous pericarditis and other forms of bacterial pericarditis in the United States is increasing as a result of the AIDS epidemic. Viral pericarditis is most commonly seen in males under 50 years of age.

### Management

Manage acute idiopathic or viral pericarditis with **bed rest and NSAIDs.** Malignant pericardial effusion can often be managed palliatively with pericardiocentesis, placement of pericardial window, radiotherapy, or chemotherapy. Purulent pericarditis requires **pericardiocentesis and IV antibiotics.** Monitor for cardiac tamponade or constrictive pericarditis. Avoid anticoagulants in light of the risk of precipitating hemorrhagic effusion.

### Complications

Complications include **cardiac tamponade and recurrences. Constrictive pericarditis** results from fibrosis of the pericardial sac, most commonly due to progression of active tuberculous pericarditis.

### Breakout Point

- Pericardial friction rub is pathognomonic
- Chest pain is worse with inspiration and lying flat, better with sitting up and leaning forward
- Most common cause is viruses
- Classic ECG finding: diffuse PR depressions and ST elevations in multiple leads

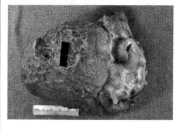

**Figure 16-3.** Shaggy, fibrinous exudate overlying the epicardial surface facing the pericardium.

# case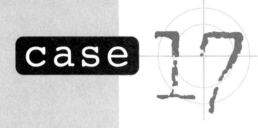

**ID/CC** A **45-year-old woman** presents with increasing **shortness of breath** over the past month.

**HPI** As a teenager, she had a prior episode of **rheumatic fever** with no known cardiac or pulmonary disease. She has recently had symptoms of **orthopnea** and several episodes of **paroxysmal nocturnal dyspnea**.

**PE** VS: normal. PE: no acute distress; lungs clear; $S_1$ (prominent) and $S_2$; mild precordial bulge; **short 2/6 diastolic murmur and 4/6 low-pitched rumbling presystolic murmur at lower left sternal border and apex with loud mid-diastolic opening snap; presystolic thrill appreciated at apex.**

**Labs** ECG: tall, peaked P-waves in limb leads and broad negative phases of diphasic P in $V_1$; right axis deviation indicating RVH.

**Imaging** CXR: enlarged left atrium; elevated left mainstem bronchus; large pulmonary artery in the presence of pulmonary hypertension. Echo: thickened, immobile mitral valve with anterior and posterior leaflets moving together.

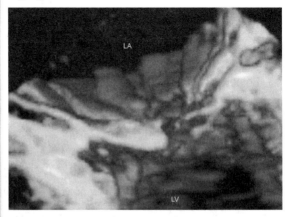

**Figure 17-1.** Echo. Thickened, immobile mitral valve with anterior and posterior leaflets moving together.

case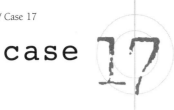

## Rheumatic Heart Disease

**Pathogenesis**

Rheumatic heart disease usually occurs as a late sequela of rheumatic fever, usually arising many years following the initial episode. The pathologic process represents an immunologic response to **streptococcal** antigens in which a **multisystem inflammatory cascade** is triggered with characteristic inflammation of the pericardium, myocardium, and endocardium. Endocarditis, valvular thickening, fibrosis, and prominent calcification occur in areas subject to greatest hemodynamic stress. The **mitral valve is most frequently involved** (50% to 60% of cases), but the aortic valve is also commonly affected (often in combination with mitral disease); tricuspid involvement is rare (<10% and almost always in association with mitral and aortic disease), and the pulmonary valve is almost never affected.

**Epidemiology**

In developed countries, the near elimination of rheumatic fever has resulted in a dramatic decrease in new cases of rheumatic heart disease. However, rheumatic heart disease continues to be prevalent in the developing world, and is also the most common underlying cause of mitral stenosis in the elderly. A history of rheumatic fever is found in only 60% of patients with rheumatic heart disease. Following the initial episode of rheumatic fever, immediate mortality is 1% to 2%; nevertheless, 80% of affected children reach adulthood, and only half have any limitation of activity secondary to valvular disease.

**Management**

Management is dependent on the specific valvular involvement. **Mitral stenosis is usually asymptomatic with minimal limitation in activity for many years. Valve replacement** is indicated in the presence of significant stenosis, insufficiency, excessive calcification, or destruction that is not amenable to valvulotomy. All patients with rheumatic heart disease should receive **prophylactic antibiotics** prior to dental, surgical, and urologic procedures to prevent endocarditis.

**Complications**

Operative mortality associated with repair procedures is low (1% to 3%). Restenosis following surgical repair may occur, but is less common with mitral valve repair. Prosthetic valve use is associated with the risk of thrombosis, paravalvular leak, endocarditis, and degenerative valvular changes.

**Breakout Point**

- Rheumatic fever occurs at ages 5 to 15 years; rheumatic heart disease occurs at ages 40 to 60 years
- "Molecular mimicry" autoimmune response to group A *Streptococcus* M antigen
- Mitral valve is most commonly affected (aortic valve is second)

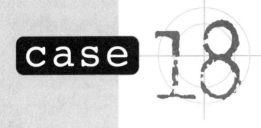

# case 18

**ID/CC** A **40-year-old woman** complains of **fever,** loss of appetite, and disabling **weakness** of 2 months' duration.

**HPI** She has been diagnosed with **rheumatic heart disease,** for which she has been receiving penicillin prophylaxis. She underwent a tooth extraction a month ago but did not take the prescribed prophylactic antibiotics. For the past 2 days, she has also had **hematuria** and a **skin rash.**

**PE** VS: fever; tachycardia. PE: ill-appearing; pallor; petechial rash over body; small, tender nodules on finger pads (OSLER NODES); tiny hemorrhages on palms and soles (JANEWAY LESIONS); clubbing of fingers; subungual **splinter hemorrhages** and conjunctival hemorrhage; oval white spots in retina (ROTH SPOTS); JVP normal; **splenomegaly;** "rumbling" mid-diastolic **murmur** with presystolic accentuation at apex; opening snap at apex (suggestive of **mitral stenosis**).

**Labs** CBC: anemia; leukocytosis. Elevated ESR. UA: proteinuria; hematuria; RBC casts. Three blood cultures taken 2 hours apart yield **viridans-group *Streptococcus.***

**Imaging** CXR, PA: superior displacement of the left main bronchus; double atrial tightening of the left heart border and pulmonary venous congestion.

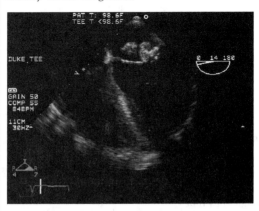

**Figure 18-1.** Transesophageal echo. Mitral valve vegetations.

# case 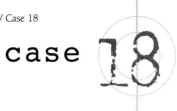18

## Subacute Bacterial Endocarditis

**Pathogenesis**

Acute endocarditis involves normal heart valves, is rapidly progressive, and is often fatal in <6 weeks. **Subacute bacterial endocarditis** (SBE) is more **chronic (>6 weeks)** and involves bacteria of relatively low virulence that are part of the normal flora. These agents are not sufficiently invasive to initiate infection in normal heart valves but may do so in **damaged or congenitally deformed valves**. More than 50% of SBE cases are caused by streptococcal species; the most common organism is *Streptococcus viridans*, which is commonly found on the **oral mucosa**. Release into the bloodstream can occur with oral manipulation; hence the need for prophylactic antibiotics prior to dental procedures. In contrast, the portal of entry for *Streptococcus bovis* usually arises from malignant or premalignant colonic lesions. **Enterococcal endocarditis** usually results from instrumentation or trauma to the lower GI or GU tract in the elderly (colonized with *Enterococcus faecalis*). HACEK organisms (*Haemophilus, Actinobacillus, Cardiobacterium, Eikenella, Kingella*) account for 5% of subacute BE cases.

**Epidemiology**

Native valve endocarditis affects males more often than females, and most patients are older than 50; the majority have a predisposing cardiac lesion. Rheumatic valvular disease accounts for 30% of cases. The mitral valve is most commonly involved, followed by the aortic valve; right-sided endocarditis is rare. Congenital heart disease other than valve prolapse (PDA, VSD, tetralogy of Fallot, coarctation of the aorta, pulmonary stenosis, and **bicuspid aortic valve**) is the underlying lesion in 10% to 20% of cases of endocarditis. Degenerative valve disease (calcific aortic stenosis in the elderly) also predisposes to infective endocarditis. No underlying heart disease is found in 20% to 40% of cases of infective endocarditis.

**Management**

High-dose **parenteral antibiotics** for 4 to 6 weeks. **Viridans streptococci** constitute the most common pathogen in SBE; **penicillin** or **penicillin plus gentamicin** is the therapy of choice. In **IV drug abusers**, suspect *Staphylococcus aureus*; treat with **nafcillin** plus gentamicin or with vancomycin if blood cultures grow methicillin-resistant *S. aureus* (MRSA). Patients with valvular disease or prosthetic heart valves should receive **antibiotic prophylaxis** prior to dental or surgical procedures.

**Complications**

Acute valvular regurgitation, pulmonary edema, and heart failure may result from valve destruction. Local spread of infection may lead to pericarditis and to aortic root or myocardial abscesses. Septic emboli may result in brain abscess or cerebritis.

**Breakout Point**

- The most common cause of acute bacterial endocarditis (normal valves): *Staphylococcus aureus*
- The most common cause of subacute bacterial endocarditis (abnormal valves): *Streptococcus viridans*

# case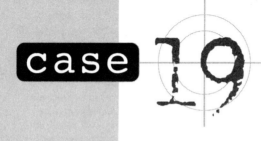

**ID/CC** A **54-year-old stockbroker** presents after suddenly fainting while eating lunch with his co-workers.

**HPI** The patient has been taking **tricyclic antidepressants** for the past 2 years. On a few occasions over the past several months, he has also experienced heaviness in the chest on exertion (ANGINA).

**PE** VS: normal. PE: alert; neurologic and cardiac exams normal.

**Labs** CBC/Lytes: normal. Calcium and glucose normal.

**Imaging** CXR: normal.

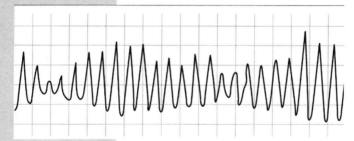

**Figure 19-1.** ECG (during episode): polymorphic ventricular tachycardia in which the axis of each successive beat changes in a characteristic "twisting of points"; QT prolongation (usually >0.6 sec).

# case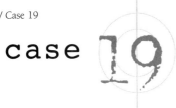

## Torsades de Pointes

**Pathogenesis**

Torsades de pointes, which literally means "twisting of points," is a specific type of ventricular tachycardia (VT) that is characterized by **polymorphic QRS complexes** that **change in amplitude and cycle length;** the syndrome is by definition associated with **QT prolongation.** Episodes of torsades de pointes are typically initiated by a premature ventricular beat occurring during a prolonged QT interval. The clinical effects depend on ventricular rate, the duration of the tachycardia, and the presence of underlying cardiac disease. Causes of acquired QT prolongation include electrolyte disturbances (hypomagnesemia, hypokalemia, hypocalcemia), drugs (quinidine, procainamide, phenothiazines, TCAs, amiodarone), and bradyarrhythmias. It may also occur as a congenital anomaly (Jervell and Lange–Nielsen syndrome, Romano–Ward syndrome) that presents primarily with cardiac arrest resulting in syncope or sudden death.

**Epidemiology**

Short-term treatment includes discontinuation of the offending agent, correction of electrolytes, IV magnesium sulfate, **beta-1 agonists in acquired long QT, temporary pacing, and** defibrillation. **Long-term treatment includes beta-blocker in congenital long QT, pacemaker implantation, and ICDs.**

**Management**

Short-term **treatment includes discontinuation of the offending agent, correction of electrolytes, IV magnesium sulfate,** beta-1 agonists in acquired long QT, temporary pacing, and **defibrillation.** Long-term treatment includes beta-blocker in congenital long QT, pacemaker implantation, and ICDs.

**Complications**

Patients with uniform VT without heart disease have a good prognosis and a low probability of sudden death. Polymorphic VT preceded by QT prolongation (>0.6 sec) may predispose patients to multiple episodes of **nonsustained VT** (<30 sec or 10 beats) with **recurrent syncope.** However, these patients may also develop ventricular fibrillation and sudden death.

**Breakout Point**

- QRS morphology "twists" around the baseline
- Most common causes are hypokalemia, hypomagnesemia, QT prolongation
- Can degenerate into ventricular tachycardia

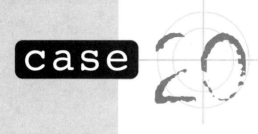

**case 20**

| | |
|---|---|
| **ID/CC** | A **58-year-old woman** complains of **intermittent chest discomfort over the last 2 hours.** |
| **HPI** | She describes **chest pressure that radiates to the shoulder and jaw** and that started at rest. She has a history of intermittent chest pain, but always elicited by exertion and relieved by rest in the past. She has a prior history of myocardial infarction requiring percutaneous coronary intervention, hypertension, and type II diabetes mellitus. |
| **PE** | VS: normal. PE: normal. |
| **Labs** | Cardiac biomarkers (CK, CK-MB, troponin I): normal. CBC/Lytes: normal. |
| **Imaging** | CXR: normal. ECG: 1-mm ST depressions in inferior leads. |

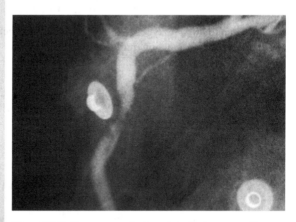

**Figure 20-1.** Coronary angiogram. Impaired coronary flow, midcoronary stenosis, and protruding thrombus downstream.

# case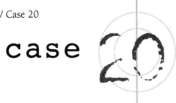

## Unstable Angina

**Pathogenesis**

Unstable angina is a **clinical syndrome** characterized by chest discomfort or anginal equivalent secondary to cardiac ischemia that is **new-onset, occurring at rest, worsening in frequency or intensity, or occurring after MI.** ECG changes including ST depressions, T-wave inversions, or ST elevations may accompany symptoms. **Negative cardiac biomarkers** suggest an absence of myocardial necrosis and distinguish unstable angina from non–ST-elevation MI and ST-elevation MI. Etiologies include nonocclusive thrombus, coronary spasm, inflammation, increased myocardial oxygen demand, or mechanical obstruction of coronary blood flow.

**Epidemiology**

Nearly 1 million patients are hospitalized each year with unstable angina. Risk factor include: age >60, hypertension, hypercholesterolemia, diabetes mellitus, smoking history, family history of coronary artery disease.

**Management**

**Oxygen, aspirin, clopidogrel, beta-blocker, heparin, or low-molecular weight heparin** all play a role in the antithrombotic treatment of unstable angina. **Sublingual nitroglycerin** and longer-acting nitrates are the mainstays of symptomatic treatment. **Risk assessment** performed using a combination of clinical judgment and published risk models guides further therapy. High-risk and intermediate-risk patients may benefit from an early-invasive strategy of percutaneous coronary intervention. Low-risk patients are managed medically and evaluated with cardiac stress testing once they are symptom-free.

**Complications**

Risk of MI and death is ~5%.

**Breakout Point**

- Acute coronary syndrome includes unstable angina, non–ST-elevation MI (NSTEMI), and ST-elevation MI (STEMI)
- Negative cardiac biomarkers, with or without ECG changes
- Presents as an acute change in anginal equivalent

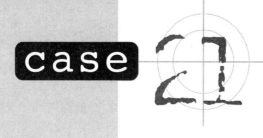

# case 21

ID/CC    A **32-year-old man** complains of frequent **palpitations**.

HPI    He denies chest pain, syncope, or dizziness.

PE    VS: HR250

Labs    See Figure 21-1.

Imaging    None.

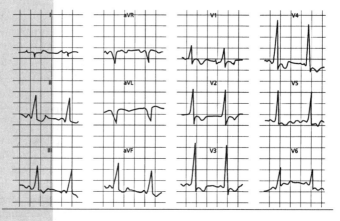

**Figure 21-1.** ECG. Shortened PR interval; slurred upstroke (DELTA WAVE); widening of QRS complex (>0.12 sec).

case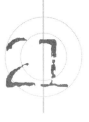

## Wolff–Parkinson–White Syndrome

**Pathogenesis**

Wolff–Parkinson–White (WPW) syndrome is a congenital abnormality involving the presence of **abnormal conductive tissue between the atria and ventricles,** often associated with SVT. The impulse is typically conducted anterograde over the normal AV system and retrograde through congenital aberrant tissue. This produces a tachycardia with a wide QRS complex with a classic delta wave (Slurred upstroke to the QRS). Most cases are asymptomatic, with evidence of preexcitation on a screening ECG. WPW syndrome can be associated with Ebstein anomaly, mitral valve prolapse, idiopathic dilated cardiomyopathy, or hypertrophic cardiomyopathy. Different types of arrhythmias occur in association with WPW syndrome: AV reentrant tachycardia (80%), atrial fibrillation (15% to 30%), and atrial flutter (5%).

**Epidemiology**

WPW syndrome is the most common type of ventricular preexcitation.

**Management**

Only treat symptomatic cases. The three main treatment modalities are drug therapy, electrical ablation, and surgical ablation. Ablation is the first-line treatment for symptomatic WPW syndrome. **Calcium-channel blockers** or **adenosine** may be used to terminate an episode of reciprocal tachycardia. **IV lidocaine or procainamide** may be used to slow the ventricular response in severe tachycardia. **Quinidine, procainamide, amiodarone,** and **sotalol** increase the refractoriness of the AV node/ bypass tract and may be used prophylactically, either empirically or based on serial electrophysiologic drug testing. If hemodynamically unstable, treat with synchronized electrical cardioversion. Digoxin is contraindicated in WPW syndrome, as it may increase conduction through the aberrant pathway.

**Complications**

Atrial fibrillation occurs commonly; rarely, ventricular arrhythmia may occur. Early recurrence of preexcitation may occur after a successful catheter ablation. Late recurrence is uncommon; sudden death is rare.

**Breakout Point**

- ECG findings: short PR interval, delta wave, wide QRS
- Congenital AV accessory pathway
- Ablation—treatment of choice

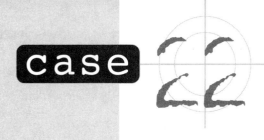

**ID/CC** A **30-year-old man** complains of increasing **weakness** and **fatigue** of 2 years' duration.

**HPI** He also states that he has been feeling **depressed,** with episodes of dizziness. He reports significant anorexia and weight loss over the past year with nearly constant **nausea.** His wife has noticed that he has become excessively irritable and restless.

**PE** VS: hypotension (BP 80/50). PE: **diffuse dark-brown hyperpigmentation** noted, especially about the elbows and skin creases; oral mucosa reveals bluish-black hyperpigmented patches.

**Labs** CBC: normocytic anemia; eosinophilia. **ACTH stimulation test** results in a **subnormal rise in cortisol.** Lytes: **hyperkalemia;** hyponatremia; hypercalcemia. ABGs: mild metabolic acidosis. Hypoglycemia.

**Imaging** CXR: normal (to check for tuberculosis).

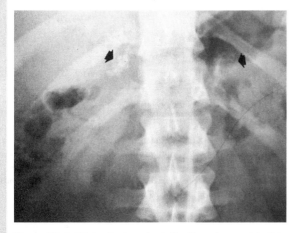

**Figure 22-1.** Bilateral adrenal calcifications (*arrows*) in this patient with tuberculous adrenal disease, causing adrenocortical insufficiency (Addison disease).

43

# case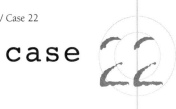

## Addison Disease

**Pathogenesis**

Primary adrenal insufficiency, or Addison disease, has two main origins: **granulomatous infections** such as TB and histoplasmosis (responsible for a minority of cases in the United States), and more commonly, **idiopathic atrophy,** which is believed to be due to an **autoimmune mechanism.** It may occur alone or as part of a polyglandular autoimmune syndrome type 1 (with mucocutaneous candidiasis and hypoparathyroidism) or type 2 (with type 1 diabetes and Hashimoto thyroiditis or Graves disease). Adrenal insufficiency can also present as part of a hereditary disorder marked by progressive myelin degeneration in the brain (adrenoleukodystrophy) or the spinal cord (adrenomyelodystrophy). Infiltration of the adrenals by opportunistic pathogens (e.g., CMV, *Cryptococcus*) and by Kaposi sarcoma may manifest as adrenal insufficiency in AIDS patients. Metastasis to the adrenals and disseminated meningococcal infection (Waterhouse–Friderichsen syndrome) are other causes of Addison disease; drugs such as ketoconazole and etomidate may also cause adrenal insufficiency. In contrast to primary adrenal insufficiency, **secondary adrenal insufficiency** (hypothalamic or pituitary insufficiency, therapeutic use of corticosteroids) **is characterized by low levels of ACTH,** and is most often due to abrupt cessation of chronic glucocorticoid treatment.

**Epidemiology**

Primary adrenocortical insufficiency is relatively rare, may occur at any age, and affects both sexes equally; because of the increasing therapeutic use of steroids, secondary adrenal insufficiency is now relatively common.

**Management**

Treatment should include both glucocorticoids and mineralocorticoids. Monitor by watching for weight gain or hypokalemia. Increase the **steroid** dosage in periods of increased stress. Addisonian crisis (hypotension, hypoglycemia, hyperkalemia) requires IV hydrocortisone, IV glucose, and aggressive IV hydration. Hydrocortisone must be given before thyroxine when hypothyroidism and Addison disease coexist (SCHMIDT SYNDROME) to prevent exacerbation of adrenal insufficiency by thyroid hormone. Provide patient with medical alert bracelet and instruct on usage of emergency IM hydrocortisone.

**Complications**

Addisonian crisis.

**Breakout Point**

- Primary adrenal insufficiency = ↑ACTH, ↓cortisol after ACTH challenge
- Secondary adrenal insufficiency = ↓ACTH, ↑cortisol after ACTH challenge
- Most common etiology is autoimmune destruction of adrenals

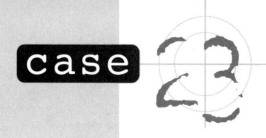

| | |
|---|---|
| **ID/CC** | A **29-year-old woman** presents with **hypertension**. |
| **HPI** | Patient found to have elevated blood pressure at her routine annual examination. On further questioning, she has had a mild headache for the last few weeks, as well as muscle aches and fatigue. |
| **PE** | VS: hypertension (BP 180/110). PE: no peripheral edema. |
| **Labs** | Lytes: **hypernatremic, hypokalemic.** ABG: mild metabolic alkalosis. **Low plasma renin level, with high plasma aldosterone-to-renin ratio.** Plasma aldosterone level does not decline with administration of normal saline. ECG: U-waves. |
| **Imaging** | CT of the abdomen: adrenal adenoma. |

ENDOCRINOLOGY

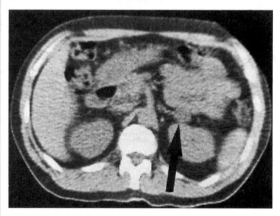

**Figure 23-1.** CT abdomen. Small mass (*arrow*) anterior to the left kidney.

# case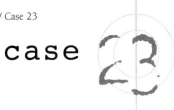

## Conn syndrome

**Pathogenesis**

Primary hyperaldosteronism results from the **autonomous production of aldosterone by the adrenal gland, in the absence of renin stimulation**. The syndrome is secondary to a **unilateral adrenal adenoma** in 60% of cases (Conn syndrome), and bilateral adrenal hyperplasia in the majority of the rest. Aldosterone acts on the distal nephron to increase sodium reabsorption in exchange for potassium and hydrogen ions. Consequently, **hypertension, hypernatremia, hypokalemia,** and a mild metabolic alkalosis ensue. In a patient presenting with hypertension and hypokalemia, primary hyperaldosteronism must be distinguished from secondary hyperaldosteronism. **Secondary hyperaldosteronism** results from **elevated plasma renin**, as seen in any state with compromised renal blood flow (renal artery stenosis, cirrhosis, and dehydration, among others). **Primary hyperaldosteronism** typically demonstrates a **low level of plasma renin**. Additional support for a primary process is provided by failure to suppress aldosterone secretion with a saline challenge. Once primary hyperaldosteronism has been confirmed, adenoma must be distinguished from bilateral adrenal hyperplasia. This is most often accomplished via CT scan or MRI of the abdomen.

**Epidemiology**

More common in women than men, with peak incidence in the third through sixth decades. One percent to three percent of patients with hypertension have Conn syndrome.

**Management**

**Surgery** is the preferred therapy for a unilateral adrenal adenoma. Use of a mineralocorticoid receptor antagonist, such as spironolactone, is an alternative for patients who cannot tolerate surgery, and is the treatment of choice for bilateral adrenal hyperplasia.

**Breakout Point**

- Primary hyperaldosteronism = ↑aldosterone, ↓renin, ↑aldosterone:renin ratio
- Secondary hyperaldosteronism = ↑aldosterone, ↑renin
- Most common etiology of primary hyperaldosteronism is a unilateral adrenal adenoma (Conn syndrome)
- Presents as hypertension, hypernatremia, hypokalemia

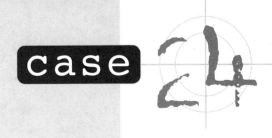

| | |
|---|---|
| **ID/CC** | A 40-year-old woman presents with **generalized muscle weakness** and **easy bruising**. |
| **HPI** | She also reports increased appetite, significant **weight gain**, and **purplish marks** over her abdomen. The patient has been amenorrheic for the past 4 months and complains of depression and inability to sleep adequately. She also complains of **increased hair growth**. |
| **PE** | VS: mild hypertension (BP 150/90). PE: acne; hirsutism; **"moon facies"**; **central obesity** with peripheral wasting; **purple striae** on abdomen; **"buffalo hump"**; **proximal muscle weakness** present. |
| **Labs** | Mildly elevated glucose. Lytes: hypokalemia; hypernatremia; metabolic alkalosis. Serum cortisol level high; **24-hour urinary free cortisol elevated; partial cortisol suppression by high-dose dexamethasone test** is consistent with pituitary ACTH excess (CUSHING DISEASE). |
| **Imaging** | MR, head (with contrast): microadenoma in the pituitary. |

ENDOCRINOLOGY

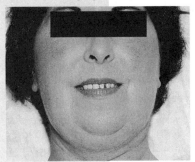

**Figure 24-1.** Characteristic "moon facies."

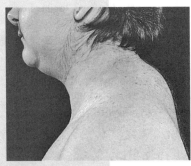

**Figure 24-3.** "Buffalo hump."

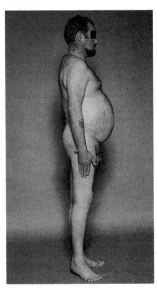

**Figure 24-2.** Central obesity with peripheral wasting.

# case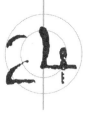

## Cushing Disease

**Pathogenesis**

Cushing **disease** is caused by increased production of ACTH by a **pituitary adenoma,** resulting in bilateral adrenal hyperplasia and excessive cortisol. Cushing **syndrome** is caused by a heterogeneous group of disorders that lead to excess cortisol through ectopic ACTH production (small-cell lung cancer, carcinoid syndrome), through primary adrenal disorders (adrenocortical adenoma, nodular hyperplasia), or through exogenous, iatrogenic causes.

**Epidemiology**

Cushing disease is most common in women of reproductive age. In the United States, most cases of Cushing syndrome are due to exogenous administration of glucocorticoids. Endogenous Cushing syndrome is rare.

**Management**

**Transsphenoidal microadenomectomy** is the treatment of choice; if pituitary imaging has identified a microadenoma, cure rates are excellent. Surgical removal is the treatment of choice for ectopic ACTH-producing tumors. Pharmacologic treatment of Cushing syndrome with agents that inhibit steroidogenesis (ketoconazole, mitotane, metyrapone) is limited to the control of extreme manifestations before surgery, supplementation of a partial remission induced by pituitary irradiation, or inoperable patients.

**Complications**

**Nelson syndrome** develops in 10% to 20% of patients after bilateral adrenalectomy. The syndrome is characterized by dramatic hyperpigmentation and by the development of a chromophobe tumor of the pituitary gland. Diabetes, infection, osteoporosis, avascular necrosis of the femoral head, thromboembolism, peripheral vascular disease, and ischemic heart disease may result from Cushing syndrome.

**Breakout Point**

- Most common etiology is iatrogenic
- Cushing disease: ↑ACTH from pituitary adenoma
- Cushing syndrome: state of hypercortisolism
- Presents as moon facies, buffalo hump, central obesity, striae, easy bruisability

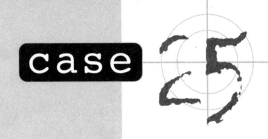

# case 25

| | |
|---|---|
| **ID/CC** | A **40-year-old woman** complains of increasing **urinary frequency** with **large volumes of urine.** |
| **HPI** | These symptoms have developed gradually over several months. She has also been **drinking more fluids.** She feels well otherwise. She specifically denies any headaches, visual changes, dizziness, weakness, numbness, or paresthesias. |
| **PE** | VS are normal. Mucous membranes are slightly dry. Neurologic examination is nonfocal. |
| **Labs** | Plasma **sodium level is high-normal.** Urine specific gravity and urine osmolality are both very low. Serum glucose is normal. |
| **Imaging** | MRI of sella: normal. |

ENDOCRINOLOGY

# case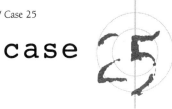

## Diabetes Insipidus

**Pathogenesis**

Diabetes insipidus (DI) can be divided into two types: central and nephrogenic. Central DI is characterized by **decreased secretion of antidiuretic hormone** (ADH). Nephrogenic DI is characterized by **resistance to the action of ADH** in the kidney. ADH determines free water excretion in the kidney by changing the permeability of the collecting tubules to water. Therefore, both central and nephrogenic DI result in a **decreased ability of the kidney to concentrate urine,** causing polyuria and polydipsia. Central DI is often **idiopathic** (possibly an autoimmune mechanism) but can also result from trauma, pituitary surgery, or hypoxic or ischemic injury. Nephrogenic DI can be due to inherited defects, **lithium use, hypercalcemia,** or chronic renal insufficiency. Patients with a nontraumatic etiology of DI can have an indolent course. If patients do not have access to adequate fluids, or if thirst is impaired, **hypernatremia and neurologic symptoms may develop.**

**Management**

If a normal thirst mechanism is present, patients can often drink enough fluids to replace urinary losses. In the case of central DI, **desmopressin** (dDAVP) is the drug of choice to replace the ADH that is lacking. If an intracranial mass is causing central DI, surgical intervention may be necessary. Nephrogenic DI can be treated with a low salt diet and thiazide diuretics (the hypovalencies induces and increase in proximal sodium and water reabsorption, decreasing water delivery to the ADH–sensitive collecting tubules).

**Breakout Point**

- Central DI: deficient secretion of ADH
- Nephrogenic DI: normal ADH secretion but renal resistance to ADH
- Central DI can be treated with exogenous ADH (desmopressin); nephrogenic cannot
- With intact thirst and access to water, hypernatremia and neurologic complications can be avoided

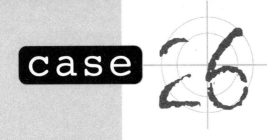

# case 26

| | |
|---|---|
| **ID/CC** | A **20-year-old white man** presents with **lethargy** that has worsened over the past 24 hours. |
| **HPI** | The patient's parents state that their son has complained of **increased thirst, frequent urination**, and **weight loss** (despite increased appetite) over the past several weeks. They add that he complained of **abdominal pain** today and had one episode of **emesis**. |
| **PE** | VS: no fever; normal BP; **elevated RR** (RR 25). PE: **thin** and **lethargic;** oriented ×3; dry mucous membranes and poor skin turgor; **fruity smell on breath** (due to ketones); **rapid, deep breathing** (KUSSMAUL RESPIRATION); abdomen soft, diffusely tender to palpation, and nondistended. |
| **Labs** | Lytes: **hyponatremia** (133 mEq/L); hyperkalemia (5.8 mEq/L); hyperchloremia (115 mEq/L); **decreased bicarbonate** (6 mEq/L). Elevated BUN and creatinine; **elevated glucose** (400 mg/dL). ABGs: **acidemia** (pH 7.15). UA: **ketonuria** and **glucosuria**. |
| **Imaging** | None. |

# case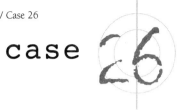

## Diabetes Mellitus, Type 1

**Pathogenesis**

The etiology of type 1 diabetes mellitus (DM) is currently unknown; however, it is known to be associated with **HLA-DR3 and -DR4,** and the destructive process affecting the pancreas is thought to be **autoimmune** in nature. Circulating islet cell antibodies and GAD antibodies have been detected in as many as 85% of patients. Environmental factors may also play a role, including viral infections. Sometimes, after the presenting ketoacidotic state, no treatment is required for a period of time (HONEYMOON PERIOD). Eventually, there is inadequate pancreatic insulin production, creating the need for insulin injections. Persistent hyperglycemia causes many of the chronic conditions associated with type 1 DM as a result of nonenzymatic glycosylation, protein deposition, and the conversion of glucose to sorbitol.

**Epidemiology**

Type 1 DM appears in 0.2% to 0.5% of the population, and occurs more commonly in whites (peak incidence at age 14). Although <10% of first-degree relatives of the proband are affected, the **concordance rate is approximately 50% with identical twins.**

**Management**

Acute management of a presenting ketoacidotic state includes IV insulin, aggressive hydration, correction of electrolyte imbalance, and treatment of any underlying precipitating cause (e.g., antibiotics for infection). Subsequently, exogenous insulin injections or insulin pump infusions are required for treatment. **Tightly regulated glucose** levels decrease the incidence and progression of complications. Patients should receive dietary **education,** regular glucose monitoring, and periodic glycosylated hemoglobin (HbA1C) monitoring (measure of glucose control over past 3 months).

**Complications**

Acutely, patients may develop **diabetic ketoacidosis (as in this case) or hypoglycemic coma.** Long-term hyperglycemia predisposes to **diabetic nephropathy, neuropathy, retinopathy, vascular disease** (peripheral disease and CAD), nonhealing wounds, and chronic infections.

**Breakout Point**

- 3 Ps: polyuria, polydipsia, polyphagia
- Autoimmune destruction of pancreatic beta-cells
- Patients require lifelong insulin
- DKA is a common complication

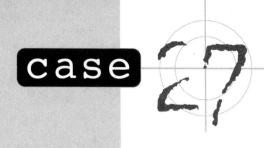

# case 27

| | |
|---|---|
| **ID/CC** | A **50-year-old man** complains of **polyuria**. |
| **HPI** | He additionally notes excessive thirst **(polydipsia)** and blurring of his vision. He has noted a gradual weight gain over years; however, more recently has been losing weight despite increased appetite. |
| **PE** | VS: hypertension (BP 142/85). PE: obese. **Cotton-wool spots** (areas of yellowish-white discoloration on the retina) and retinal **microaneurysms** on ophthalmoscopy. Hyperpigmentation over axillary creases. Decreased proprioception in feet. |
| **Labs** | Fasting plasma glucose 165 mg/dL. Urinalysis: protein and glucose present. Urine albumin-to-creatinine ratio >30 mg/mmol (such a ratio is indicative of proteinuria, which is commonly seen in conditions such as poorly controlled diabetes or hypertension). |
| **Imaging** | None. |

ENDOCRINOLOGY

# case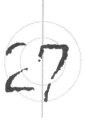

## Diabetes Mellitus, Type 2

**Pathogenesis**

The pathogenesis of diabetes mellitus type 2 is thought to involve both **deranged insulin secretion** and **insulin resistance.** Resultant hyperglycemia promotes **nonenzymatic glycosylation,** whereby glucose attaches to proteins, causing alterations in protein function and, ultimately, organ damage. The major complications are vascular, including **atherosclerosis** (large vessel involvement, such as the coronary arteries), and **microangiopathy** (small vessel involvement, such as the glomeruli, vasa nervosum, and retinal vessels, leading to **nephropathy, neuropathy,** and **retinopathy**). The neuropathy is most commonly sensorimotor, in a **stocking-glove** distribution. The diagnosis is made by demonstration of one of the following:

- Symptoms *and* random plasma glucose level >200 mg/dL *or*
- Fasting plasma glucose level >126 mg/dL *or*
- Two-hour plasma glucose level >200 mg/dL during an oral glucose-tolerance test

**Epidemiology**

Affects more than 15 million people in the United States. Most patients are >50 years old, and 80% are obese. Carries a strong genetic basis. **Myocardial infarction** is the most common cause of death, and can be silent.

**Management**

The cornerstones of management are **lifestyle and dietary modification.** Initially, most can be managed with an oral agent alone, such as an insulin sensitizer (a **biguanide,** or a **thiazolidinedione**), or an insulin secretagogue (a **sulfonylurea,** or a **meglitinide**). Insulin secretagogues pose the risk of hypoglycemia. Eventually, many require insulin therapy. The goal hemoglobin A1c is <7%. Consider an angiotensin-converting-enzyme inhibitor in those with microalbuminuria.

**Complications**

**Hyperosmolar nonketotic coma** may result from sustained hyperglycemia leading to severe dehydration. Management requires aggressive fluid and electrolyte repletion. Diabetics are also more prone to **infection,** and have **impaired wound healing.**

**Breakout Point**

- Obese patients
- Strong genetic basis

### ■ TABLE 27-1 OTHER THERAPEUTIC GOALS IN TYPE 2 DIABETES

Aglycosuria
Freedom from symptoms
Normalize plasma total cholesterol
Normalize plasma LDL cholesterol
Normalize plasma triglycerides
Normalize blood pressure
Smoking cessation
Body weight stable and as close to normal as possible

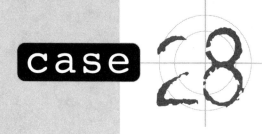

case 28

**ID/CC**  A **25-year-old man** is brought to the emergency room in a **comatose state.**

**HPI**  He has been diagnosed with **insulin-dependent diabetes mellitus (IDDM)** and has been receiving insulin for 6 years. His parents report three similar incidents in the past, each preceded by **urinary frequency, nausea, and vomiting.**

**PE**  VS: tachycardia (HR 110). PE: comatose and moderately dehydrated; Kussmaul breathing noted.

**Labs**  Lytes: potassium initially elevated (hydration and correction of acidosis invariably lower serum levels, unmasking profound total body depletion); hyponatremia. Serum glucose elevated. ABGs: **anion-gap acidosis.** Elevated levels of **ketone bodies** (acetoacetate, $\beta$-hydroxybutyrate, acetone) in urine and serum.

**Imaging**  None.

case

## Diabetic Ketoacidosis

**Pathogenesis**

The two cardinal features of diabetic ketoacidosis (DKA)—**acidosis** and **hyperglycemia**—are caused by the combined effects of severe insulin deficiency and excessive secretion of counterregulatory hormones such as glucagon, which interact synergistically to potentiate the effects of insulin loss. These changes mobilize the delivery of substrates from muscle (amino acids, lactate, pyruvate) and adipose tissue (free fatty acids, glycerol) to the liver, where they are actively converted to glucose (via gluconeogenesis) or ketone bodies (β-hydroxybutyrate, acetoacetate). The net result is **hyperglycemia** (>300 mg%), anion-gap metabolic **acidosis** (pH <7.35), and an osmotic diuresis that leads to marked **dehydration**. Hyponatremia results from increased plasma osmolality from excessive serum glucose that pulls water out of cells, decreasing sodium concentration by dilution.

**Epidemiology**

DKA may herald the onset of type 1 IDDM but occurs most often in previously diagnosed diabetic patients as a result of intercurrent illness, emotional stress, or inadequate insulin administration.

**Management**

**IV insulin; ample IV fluids** to compensate for dehydration; replete potassium and phosphate; sodium bicarbonate may be given to combat severe acidemia. Search for and treat underlying causes (e.g., infection). Insulin is required in DKA even after blood glucose normalizes—continue with insulin and glucose-containing IVF. Patients should be closely monitored for fluid overload cerebral edema, hypo-or hyperkalemia.

**Complications**

**Impaired cardiac and respiratory function** secondary to acidemia may reduce ventricular threshold to fibrillation. **Mortality** remains approximately 10%.

**Breakout Point**

- Anion-gap metabolic acidosis
- Production of ketone bodies: acetoacetate, B-hydroxybutyrate
- Life-threatening condition
- Common complication of type 1 but not type 2 diabetes

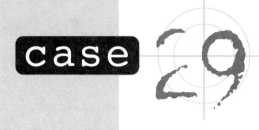

**case 29**

**ID/CC** A **44-year-old woman** complains of a **painful rash on her face, abdomen, distal extremities, and perineum** (MIGRATORY NECROLYTIC ERYTHEMA).

**HPI** The patient frequently drinks large amounts of fluid, urinates often, including twice during the night, and eats voraciously (POLYDIPSIA, POLYURIA, AND POLYPHAGIA OF DIABETES MELLITUS). Nevertheless, she acknowledges a **weight loss** of approximately 25 kg in the last year. She also states that she frequently feels lethargic and tires easily (secondary to anemia).

**PE** VS: normal. PE: **rash appears erythematous, raised, and scaly** with presence of bullae and crusting; scleral icterus (secondary to hepatic metastases); **glossitis; dystrophic nails; thinning hair.**

**Labs** CBC: low hematocrit (29%). Glucose elevated; abnormal glucose tolerance test; **fasting plasma glucagon elevated** (>1,000 pg/mL); total cholesterol low. LFTs: normal.

**Imaging** CT, abdomen: lobulated mass in the tail of the pancreas with extension into the superior mesenteric vein; solitary, metastatic lesion in the right lobe of the liver.

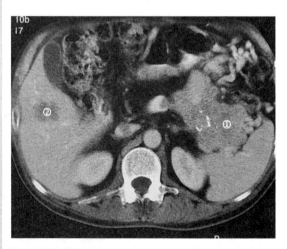

**Figure 29-1.** CT, abdomen. Lobulated mass (*1*) in the tail of the pancreas with extension into the superior mesenteric vein; solitary, metastatic lesion (*2*) in the right lobe of the liver.

# case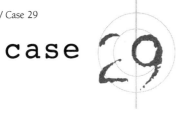

## Glucagonoma

**Pathogenesis**

Glucagonomas are **malignant pancreatic ($\alpha_2$) islet cell tumors that primarily secrete glucagon** as well as other peptides, such as gastrin, insulin, somatostatin, and pancreatic polypeptide (at lower levels). They are characterized by the presence of diabetes mellitus, necrolytic migratory erythema, anemia, and weight loss. These tumors may also rarely present in the context of MEN type I (WERMER SYNDROME), and are generally biologically inactive in this context.

**Epidemiology**

These tumors are generally **rare, solitary, and slow-growing,** and approximately 50% **present with metastatic disease, usually to the liver or bone.**

**Management**

Optimal management is **operative resection;** this is the only curative therapy. Even if eradication is not possible, surgical debulking prolongs survival and provides effective palliation. Currently, active drugs used to treat glucagonomas do not exist, although some drugs can cause partial regression of the mass or improvement in the symptoms of MNE. These drugs include doxorubicin, streptozotocin, and octreotide. Chemotherapeutic regimens are of little benefit. Hepatic artery embolization may provide some relief.

**Complications**

Liver and bone metastases.

**Breakout Point**

- Presents as diarrhea, peptic ulcer, necrolytic migratory erythema
- Usually malignant

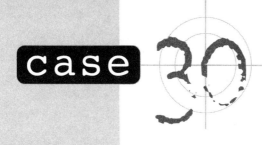

# case

**ID/CC** A **30-year-old woman** complains of **anxiety, diaphoresis, palpitations, and inability to concentrate** over the past 2 months.

**HPI** She also has had **blurry vision, irregular menses, and a 10-lb unintentional weight loss** over the past month. Her boyfriend states that she has been emotionally labile and has only been sleeping 3 hours a night.

**PE** VS: low-grade fever, tachycardic. PE: thyroid gland is **diffusely enlarged without tenderness; proptosis** is observed; raised, hyperpigmented, **orange-peel textured papules** are noted over the bilateral shins; skin is warm and moist; hands have a fine tremor.

**Labs** CBC: normocytic anemia, mild leukocytosis with WBC of 12. Glucose: normal. **TSH: high. Free T4: undetectable.**

**Imaging** Nuclear Thyroid Scan: **diffuse uptake throughout the thyroid gland.** ECG: sinus tachycardia.

ENDOCRINOLOGY

case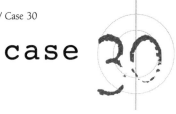

## Graves Disease

**Pathogenesis**

Graves disease is an autoimmune disorder that causes hyperthyroidism. **Autoantibodies known as thyroid-stimulating immunoglobulins (TSIs) activate the TSH receptor,** mimicking the function of TSH itself. Graves disease is characterized by **ophthalmopathy** (proptosis and periorbital edema) and **pretibial myxedema.** These clinical manifestations are felt to be immune mediated.

**Epidemiology**

Graves disease has an incidence of approximately 1% of the population and affects primarily those aged 20 to 40. Women are affected 7 times more than men. Predisposing factors are genetics, smoking, recent pregnancy, and iodine-containing medications such as amiodarone.

**Management**

Goals of treatment focus on inhibiting thyroid hormone synthesis, blocking peripheral conversion of T4 to T3 (active thyroid hormone), and blocking the peripheral effects. Treatment should include **thionamides such as propylthiouracil and methimazole.** Propylthiouracil inhibits new thyroid hormone synthesis and peripheral conversion of T4 to T3 (active thyroid hormone). Methimazole inhibits new thyroid hormone synthesis, but not peripheral conversion. **Beta-blockers (such as propranolol)** are the mainstay of symptomatic therapy by decreasing peripheral conversion and by decreasing sympathetic hyperactivity. **Iodides, such as Lugol Solution,** can block release of preformed thyroid hormone.

**Complications**

**Thyroid storm** is characterized by a large release of thyroid hormones that creates a life-threatening condition. Clinical manifestations include fever, tachycardia, abdominal pain, and neurologic complications.

**Breakout Point**

- Anti-TSH receptor autoantibodies activate the TSH receptor
- Causes exophthalmos and proptosis

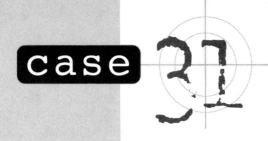

# case

**ID/CC** A **45-year-old woman** presents with **generalized swelling of the neck** that has progressively worsened over the past 2 years.

**HPI** She also has a history of chronic **constipation, cold intolerance,** skin coarseness, edema, headaches, weight gain, arthralgias, **hoarseness, fatigue,** and prior carpal tunnel surgery.

**PE** VS: **bradycardia.** PE: coarse, dry skin; nonpitting **pedal edema;** midline goiter moves with deglutition; goiter rubbery with enlarged pyramidal lobe; no cervical lymphadenopathy noted.

**Labs** Depressed $T_3$ and $T_4$; elevated TSH; high antithyroid peroxidase (TPO) antibody titers; high antithyroglobulin antibody titers. FNA: lymphocytic and plasma cell infiltration of gland tissue.

**Imaging** None.

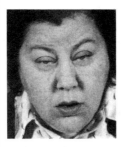

**Figure 31-1.** Characteristic facies with the facial and periorbital swelling.

# case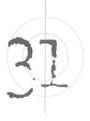

## Hashimoto Thyroiditis

**Pathogenesis**

Demonstration of elevated **antithyroid antibodies** and **lymphocytic infiltration** of the thyroid gland **with destruction of the thyroid cells** in Hashimoto thyroiditis underscores the autoimmune basis of its etiology. Inflammation may initially produce hyperthyroidism followed by a period of euthyroidism before the disease progresses. As the inflammatory process progressively destroys thyroid tissue, partial or severe hypothyroidism results. The presence of copious lymphocytes is a hallmark of the disease that distinguishes it from other forms of autoimmune thyroiditis.

**Epidemiology**

Hashimoto thyroiditis is the most common cause of primary hypothyroidism in the United States after the age of 6 years. The most common cause of hypothyroidism worldwide is iodine deficiency in areas of inadequate iodine intake. The incidence is 10 to 15 times **more common in women** and is most frequently diagnosed between the third and fifth decades of life. A genetic propensity for the disease is demonstrated by an increased familial incidence and an association with MHC antigens such as HLA-B8.

**Management**

**Thyroxine** replacement is used indefinitely to suppress the goiter or to correct hypothyroidism (monitor TSH). Indications for surgery include obstructive goiter and malignant nodule(s).

**Complications**

Pregnant women with high antibody titers are at high risk for **miscarriage.** Hashimoto thyroiditis commonly coexists with other autoimmune diseases, including pernicious anemia, Sjögren syndrome, Graves disease, SLE, adrenal insufficiency, and diabetes mellitus. Myxedema coma is a state of extreme hypothyroidism and is associated with high mortality.

**Breakout Point**

| Most Common Cause of Primary Hypothyroidism |
|---|
| • High antithyroid peroxidase and antithyroglobulin antibodies |
| • ↑TSH, ↓T4, ↑T3 |

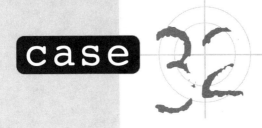

# case 32

**ID/CC** A **55-year-old woman** complains of **nausea, vomiting, constipation, abdominal pain**, thirst, and frequent urination.

**HPI** The patient states that she has not wanted to eat (ANOREXIA), has lost approximately 10 pounds in the past 2 months, and frequently feels **fatigued, weak, and depressed.** She adds that she passed a **kidney stone** approximately 1 month ago.

**PE** VS: hypertension. PE: alert and oriented ×3; hypoactive bowel sounds; **proximal muscle weakness; hyporeflexia.**

**Labs** Lytes: **elevated calcium** (12.5 mg/dL); **low phosphate** (2.0 mg/dL); elevated chloride. **PTH elevated.** UA: **hypercalciuria.** ECG: **short QT interval.**

**Imaging** XR, chest and abdomen (Figure 32-1): generalized bony demineralization with striking prominence of residual trabeculae.

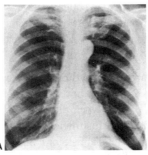

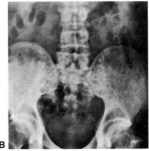

**Figure 32-1.** XR chest **(A)** and abdomen **(B).** Generalized bony demineralization with striking prominence of residual trabeculae.

case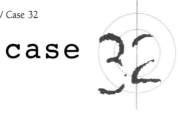

## Hyperparathyroidism—Primary

**Pathogenesis**

Primary hyperparathyroidism is characterized by **hypercalcemia** and **hypophosphatemia** secondary to **increased PTH secretion.** The causes of primary hyperparathyroidism include parathyroid adenomas (most common cause, 85% of cases), parathyroid hyperplasia (4 glands involved in 14% of cases), and parathyroid carcinomas (1% of cases). It can also be associated with MEN II and MEN III syndromes.

**Epidemiology**

**Ninety percent** of cases of **hypercalcemia** arise as a **result of hyperparathyroidism** or **malignancy.** Primary hyperparathyroidism is more prevalent in **middle-aged and elderly women.**

**Management**

**IV hydration** followed by **furosemide diuresis** to acutely lower serum calcium. **Parathyroidectomy** is the definitive treatment; commonly one of the resected parathyroid glands is implanted in the forearm for future use if the patient develops hypoparathyroidism. **Bisphosphonates** (etidronate or pamidronate) and calcitonin are used while awaiting **parathyroidectomy. Avoid thiazide diuretics.**

**Complications**

**Cardiac arrhythmias** may arise with calcium levels >12 mg/dL. Above 13 mg/dL, **metastatic calcification** (especially when phosphate is concomitantly elevated) and **renal insufficiency** may result. Above 15 mg/dL, patients are at risk for **coma and cardiac arrest.** Other complications include GI disease (pancreatitis and peptic ulcer disease), renal disease (nephrolithiasis and nephrocalcinosis), and skeletal complications (pseudogout and osteitis fibrosa cystica).

**Breakout Point**

- "Stones, bones, groans, and psychiatric overtones"
- Primary hyperparathyroidism = ↑PTH, ↑Ca, ↓Phos
- Most common cause is parathyroid adenoma

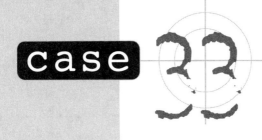

# case

**ID/CC** A **47-year-old woman** presents **following a thyroidectomy** complaining of **painful cramps and spasms in her hands** (TETANY).

**HPI** She also states that she has noticed **tingling of her hands, face, and feet** (PARESTHESIAS). She denies any history of **bone pain** or **seizures**.

**PE** VS: normal. PE: alert and oriented; tapping over facial nerve anterior to ear causes local muscle twitching (POSITIVE CHVOSTEK SIGN); tetanic carpal spasm following inflation of sphygmomanometer on arm (POSITIVE TROUSSEAU SIGN); 4/5 muscle strength in extremities; normal two-point and sharp/dull discrimination.

**Labs** **Low calcium** (7.0 mg/dL); **elevated phosphate** (5.5 mg/dL); normal magnesium; normal alkaline phosphatase; **PTH low.** ECG: **prolonged QT interval.**

**Imaging** None.

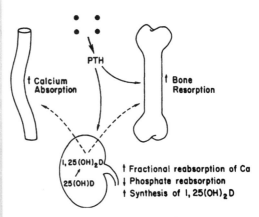

**Figure 33-1.** Effects of parathyroid hormone.

case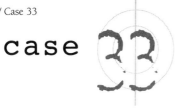

## Hypoparathyroidism

**Pathogenesis**

Acquired hypoparathyroidism is typically due to **accidental surgical removal of the parathyroid glands** (typically in patients with hyperthyroidism). Other causes include radiation-induced damage, hemochromatosis, and repeated blood transfusions.

**Epidemiology**

Most commonly due to accidental damage during neck surgery; commonly occurs transiently after thyroid surgery.

**Management**

**Calcium gluconate** by slow IV push for acutely symptomatic patients. For long-term therapy, administer **vitamin D** and **calcium.**

**Complications**

Calcification of basal ganglia leading to parkinsonian signs and symptoms; optic lens calcification leading to cataracts.

**Breakout Point**

- ↓PTH, ↑ calcium
- Parathyroids are often inadvertently removed during thyroidectomy

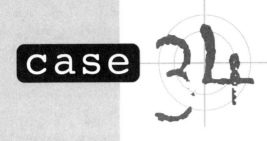

ENDOCRINOLOGY

**ID/CC**   A **50-year-old woman** complains of increasing **weakness, mental slowness,** and a progressive **increase in weight** despite a reduced appetite.

**HPI**   She also complains of wrist pain radiating to her hands as well as chronic **constipation, cold intolerance,** an increasingly husky voice (due to myxedema around vocal cords), decreased auditory acuity, and **menorrhagia.** A few years ago, she underwent a surgical thyroidectomy for Graves disease.

**PE**   VS: **bradycardia** (HR 56). PE: expressionless face; **rough, dry skin;** brittle hair; carotenemia; scar from previous **thyroidectomy** seen; Tinel sign and Phalen maneuver positive (median nerve compression/carpal tunnel syndrome); delayed relaxation of DTRs.

**Labs**   CBC: normocytic, normochromic anemia. Low total serum $T_3$ and $T_4$; **TSH elevated.** Lytes: hyponatremia (due to SIADH). ECG: bradycardia; low voltage complexes. Increased serum cholesterol.

**Imaging**   CXR: enlarged heart shadow. Echo: pericardial effusion.

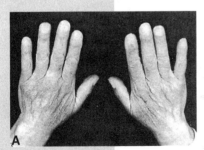
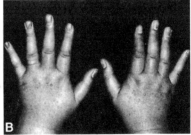

**Figure 34-1. A.** Severe dryness of the skin of the hands. **B.** Nonpitting edema of the hands of a patient with hypothyroidism.

case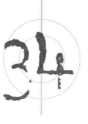

## Hypothyroidism—Primary

**Pathogenesis**

The most frequent causes of hypothyroidism are **chronic Hashimoto thyroiditis** and **ablative therapy** for hyperthyroidism. A less common cause is **neck irradiation** for cancers such as lymphoma. **Amiodarone** can cause hypothyroidism as well as hyperthyroidism; neither effect requires preexisting thyroid disease. The presence of immunoglobulins that bind to the TSH receptor but that do not stimulate thyroid function can also lead to thyroid deficiency. Finally, hypothalamic or pituitary deficiency can cause secondary hypothyroidism, but this mechanism accounts for <5% of cases.

**Epidemiology**

The incidence of hypothyroidism varies somewhat with **geographic area.** In areas with adequate iodine supply (e.g., the United States), only 0.82% to 1.0% of the population is hypothyroid; in **iodine-deficient areas,** however, the incidence is **10- to 20-fold higher.** The prevalence of hypothyroidism is **greater in females** than in males (5 in 15 versus 1 in 100).

**Management**

Synthetic **thyroid hormone replacement** (levothyroxine); treat until TSH normalizes and patient is symptom free. In patients with CAD, levothyroxine should be initiated at a low dose with small dose increments until the patient is euthyroid.

**Complications**

Myxedema coma. Hyperlipidemia and ischemic heart disease are associated with long-standing hypothyroidism. Maternal hypothyroidism during pregnancy results in offspring with IQ scores that are an average of seven points lower than those of the offspring of euthyroid mothers.

**Breakout Point**

> Hypothyroidism is the great pretender (may manifest with a wide variety of symptoms, including depression).

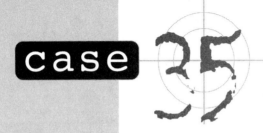

# case 35

**ID/CC** A **56-year-old** man is brought to the ER in a state of **confusion.**

**HPI** His sister states that he had previously been complaining of intermittent episodes of **slurred speech, headaches, and visual disturbances.** These episodes usually **occurred after periods of fasting** and were **alleviated by eating.**

**PE** VS: tachycardia. PE: oriented to person but not place or time; **tremulous, diaphoretic,** and **pale;** lungs clear to auscultation bilaterally.

**Labs** **Low glucose** (23 mg/dL); **serum insulin elevated; proinsulin elevated; C-peptide elevated** (rules out surreptitious insulin administration); urine screen for sulfonylurea negative; cortisol normal (rules out hypothalamic–pituitary–adrenal axis abnormality).

**Imaging** See Figures 35-1 to 35-4.

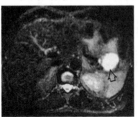

**Figure 35-1.** MR, abdomen. The inversion recovery technique shows an enhancing mass *(arrow)* in the tail of the pancreas.

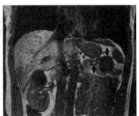

**Figure 35-2.** MR, abdomen. Before gadolinium is given, a low-signal mass *(arrow)* is seen in the tail.

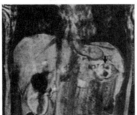

**Figure 35-3.** The mass *(arrow)* is seen to enhance after administration of gadolinium.

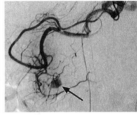

**Figure 35-4.** Angio. Another case shows a round, vascular lesion in the pancreatic head.

# case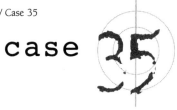

## Insulinoma

**Pathogenesis**

Insulinomas are **beta-cell neoplasms** that are located primarily in the pancreas. Increased insulin production can lead to the **Whipple triad**, which consists of **(1) symptoms of hypoglycemia, (2) fasting hypoglycemia**, and **(3) relief of symptoms with administration of IV glucose and restoration of normoglycemia.** The hypoglycemia subsequently induces catecholamine release and consequent symptoms.

**Epidemiology**

Insulinomas are **rare** tumors that generally appear in the **fifth to seventh decade as single, benign adenomas.** Ten percent are multiple and ten percent are malignant (spread to local lymph nodes and liver). They may also present in the context of MEN type I.

**Management**

Treat acutely with **IV or oral glucose.** Definitive therapy involves **surgical removal** of the adenoma or partial pancreatectomy. If surgery is not possible, patients should receive **diazoxide or octreotide** (inhibits insulin release) and streptozocin and doxorubicin (chemotherapy combination of choice for insulinoma).

**Complications**

Hypoglycemic episodes may result in trauma, brain injury, coma, or death.

**Breakout Point**

- Low C-peptide level indicates surreptitious insulin administration
- Immediate recovery with administration of glucose

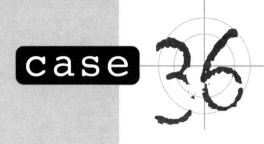

# case 36

**ID/CC** A **70-year-old man** with a prior history of **non–insulin-dependent** diabetes mellitus (NIDDM), CAD, hypertension, and glaucoma presents to the ER with complaints of increasing **lethargy over the past week.**

**HPI** He also complains of **urinary frequency** and **persistent thirst.** He has become increasingly lethargic and **confused.**

**PE** VS: supine BP normal, P 80; standing BP 98/65, P 102 (ORTHOSTATIC HYPOTENSION). PE: lethargic, uncommunicative, oriented to person only, and in mild distress; skin pale, cool, and tented; pallor; lungs clear.

**Labs** **Elevated glucose** (>600 mg/dL); **hyperosmolality** (>310 mOsm/kg). ABGs: **pH normal** (no acidosis); serum $HCO_3$ normal; normal anion gap (9 to 14 mEq/L). Elevated BUN (101 mg/dL) with normal creatinine (PRERENAL AZOTEMIA).

**Imaging** None.

ENDOCRINOLOGY

# case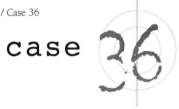

## Nonketotic Hyperosmolar Coma

**Pathogenesis**

Nonketotic hyperosmolar syndrome occurs in patients with **Type 2 diabetes mellitus** who have a **partial or relative insulin deficiency.** There is a decrease in peripheral utilization of glucose that induces glucagon secretion, which in turn stimulates hepatic gluconeogenesis. As a result of massive hyperglycemia, glucose excretion in urine increases, producing a strong osmotic diuresis. This produces **significant plasma volume contraction, dehydration,** and **reduced renal perfusion.** Renal hypoperfusion results in decreased urinary glucose loss and even higher blood glucose concentrations. Consequently, a severely hyperosmolar state develops, resulting in mental **confusion** and eventually **coma.** Because the basal requirement of insulin is not compromised, ketosis does not occur.

**Management**

**Fluid replacement** should be initiated immediately if the patient is hypovolemic. Nearly 4 to 6 L of fluid may be required in the first 8 to 10 hours. Careful monitoring of sodium and $H_2O$ replacement is important. Replace **potassium** and administer **insulin.** Once blood glucose drops to 250 mg/dL, fluid replacement should include 5% dextrose infusion that is titrated to maintain glycemic levels of 250 to 300 mg/dL. Phosphate replacement may also be needed.

**Complications**

The overall mortality of nonketotic hyperglycemic hyperosmolar coma is >10 times that of diabetic ketoacidosis primarily because of its higher incidence in older patients with significant comorbidity, as well as the delay in recognition (and treatment) of this syndrome.

**Breakout Point**

- Hyperglycemia >600 in the absence of significant ketosis (versus ketone bodies in DKA)
- Normal anion gap (versus anion gap acidosis in DKA)
- Older adults (versus younger in DKA)

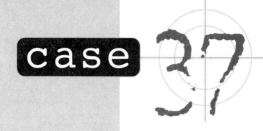

ID/CC  A **54-year-old man** from Siberia complains of **pelvic weakness** that he experiences when he rises to a standing position from a seated position.

HPI  The patient is a refugee from a Siberian prison who sought political asylum in the United States. His symptoms are associated with **bone pain** and **tenderness** in the pelvic region but are also present to a lesser extent in his spine. The patient also reports that he experienced significant weight loss secondary to **poor nutrition** during the last 2 years of his imprisonment. He was locked up in a **dark cell** with other prisoners prior to his escape.

PE  VS: normal. PE: thin and poorly nourished; localized **tenderness in pelvic girdle and spine** with moderate **decrease in proximal lower extremity motor strength.**

Labs  CBC/Lytes: normal. **Low serum calcium; low serum phosphate; increased alkaline phosphatase; low 25-hydroxyvitamin D; low urine calcium.**

Imaging  See Figures 37-1 and 37-2.

ENDOCRINOLOGY

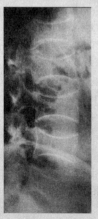

**Figure 37-1.** XR, spine. Decreased bone density and partial central collapse of all vertebral bodies.

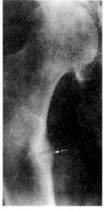

**Figure 37-2.** XR, femur. A different case shows a horizontal lucency with sclerotic margins (*arrow*; LOOSER ZONE) in the cortex of the medial femur.

case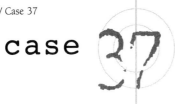

## Osteomalacia

| | |
|---|---|
| Pathogenesis | Osteomalacia is characterized by **defective mineralization of organic bone matrix that may result from inadequate dietary intake or malabsorption of vitamin D** (as in chronic pancreatitis with exocrine insufficiency), acquired or inherited disorders of vitamin D metabolism (anticonvulsant therapy, renal failure), chronic acidosis (renal tubular acidosis, acetazolamide ingestion), renal tubular defects that produce hypophosphatemia (Fanconi syndrome), and aluminum toxicity. |
| Epidemiology | Common in underdeveloped countries owing to dietary deficiency and poverty. In developed countries, it is seen with food fads or eating disorders (e.g., anorexia nervosa). Inadequate sun exposure may be seen in the elderly. Malabsorption may be seen in patients with a history of pancreatic or other GI disease, whereas defects in vitamin D metabolism may be seen in patients with liver or renal disease. Severe vitamin D deficiency is found in 3.5% of women in the United States. |
| Management | Correct the underlying cause; **supplement vitamin D, calcium, phosphate.** Radiologic evidence of recovery is seen at 1 to 6 months. Patients receiving phenytoin therapy may be treated prophylactically with vitamin D. |
| Complications | Bone pain and tenderness may develop quickly, particularly within the spine, ribs, pelvis, and lower extremities. Proximal muscle weakness is also common, especially in the lower extremities. **Fractures may occur with minimal trauma.** |
| Breakout Point | • Vitamin D deficiency in children causes rickets<br>• Vitamin D deficiency in adults causes osteomalacia |

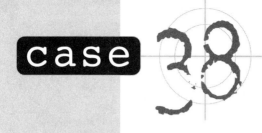

case 38

**ID/CC**  A **68-year-old white woman** presents with low **back pain.**

**HPI**  She underwent menopause when she was 52 years old. She has never taken hormone replacement therapy. She exercises regularly. She has no personal history of fractures; her mother had a hip fracture at age 79. She is a nonsmoker.

**PE**  VS: normal. PE: **loss of height** by 2 cm, weight 110 lbs, point tenderness to palpation of L-spine, **thoracic kyphosis** with "dowager's hump" (abnormal rounding of upper back).

**Labs**  **Serum calcium, phosphorus, 25-hydroxyvitamin D, alkaline phosphatase: normal.** TSH: normal.

**Imaging**  Lumbar spine films: new vertebral fracture; DEXA (dual energy x-ray absorptiometry) scan of lumbar vertebrae and hip: bone mineral density **T-score of −2.5 (low).**

ENDOCRINOLOGY

case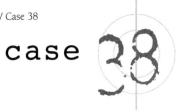

## Osteoporosis

**Pathogenesis**

**Osteoporosis** causes a range of diseases from asymptomatic bone loss to debilitating joint fractures, most common in post-menopausal women. It is characterized by **loss of bone mass** and skeletal architecture deterioration, causing increased bone fragility and risk of falls. Calcium enhances mineralization of bone; vitamin D enhances calcium absorption from the gastrointestinal tract and reabsorption in the kidneys. Risk factors include **increased age, low body weight** (<126 lbs), **maternal history of osteoporosis, history of fracture in first-degree relative, prior fractures,** current **smokers,** recent weight loss of >10 lbs, **delayed menarche (age >15), physical inactivity,** and **chronic steroid use.**

**Epidemiology**

1.5 million osteoporotic fractures per year in United States. Approximately one-half are vertebral fractures. Incidence is higher in women than men, and higher in Caucasians than African-Americans.

**Management**

Mainstays of therapy include **calcium** and **vitamin D** supplementation, and regular **weight-bearing exercise.** **Bisphosphonates** inhibit the attachment of osteoclasts to bone matrix; side effects include esophagitis. A bisphosphonate derivative, Ibandronate, may help to replace bone loss. Hormonal replacement therapy with estrogen increases bone mineral density; however, concerns about the risks of hormonal treatment (increases MI, stroke, thrombosis, and breast cancer risk) has made this option undesirable. Selective estrogen receptor modulators (SERMs) such as raloxifene have been shown to reduce the risk of vertebral fractures. **Screening of bone mineral density testing with the DEXA scan is recommended for all women >65 years of age,** and earlier for men or women with one or more risk factors as above. Bone mineral density T-score is defined as standard deviation from the mean. Nasal calcitonin is useful for decreasing pain from osteoporotic fractures.

**Complications**

Fracture.

**Breakout Point**

- Often asymptomatic, fractures discovered incidentally
- Serum PTH, calcium, phosphorus, alkaline phosphatase normal
- Treat with calcium, vitamin D, bisphosphonates, exercise

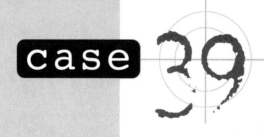

case 29

**ID/CC** A **20-year-old woman** complains of increasing episodes of **sweating, tremors,** headache, and **tachycardia** of 6 months' duration.

**HPI** She reports episodes of palpitations, weakness, and occasionally overt panic attacks over the past 2 months. Of note, when the patient presented for a cholecystectomy, she developed a hypertensive crisis complicated by an **arrhythmia during induction of anesthesia.**

**PE** VS: hypertension (BP 210/100) and tachycardia (HR120). PE: **patient is anxious, tachycardic, and diaphoretic.** Her abdominal exam shows positive bowel sounds without tenderness. Her extremities are tremulous.

**Labs** CBC: normocytic anemia. **24-hour urine metanephrines, vanillylmandelic acid, and catecholamines: increased.**

**Imaging** CT abdomen: enhancing 3-cm adrenal mass.

ENDOCRINOLOGY

# case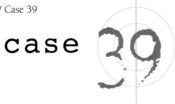

## Pheochromocytoma

**Pathogenesis**

Pheochromocytomas arise from **chromogranin cells in the adrenal medulla that secrete catecholamines.** Extra-adrenal tumors can occur anywhere along the sympathetic chain. Chromogranin A is a protein stored in neuroendocrine cells that is secreted with catecholamines; it is increased in 80% of people with pheochromocytoma, although elevations may be seen in other neuroendocrine tumors as well.

**Epidemiology**

Occurs in 0.05% to 0.2% of hypertensive individuals. Ten percent are found incidentally and 50% are diagnosed at autopsy, since patients may be completely asymptomatic. Occurs in familial syndromes, such as MEN 2A and 2B, neurofibromatosis, and von Hippel–Lindau (VHL) disease.

**Management**

**Laparoscopic adrenalectomy** for resection of pheochromocytoma is a **high-risk procedure.** In patients with known disease, alpha-adrenergic blockers and beta-blockers are started prior to surgical procedures. For acute hypertensive crisis, agents such as nitroprusside and **alpha-blockers such as phentolamine** are indicated. Lidocaine and esmolol may be used to control cardiac arrhythmias. Ten percent of catecholamine-secreting tumors are malignant. Chemotherapeutic regimens are beneficial but not curative. Monitoring should be long term, with annual biochemical screening even in patients who appear cured. Screening for inherited diseases should be performed because this tumor is present in MEN 2A and 2B, neurofibromatosis, and VHL syndrome.

**Complications**

In patients with an undiagnosed tumor, undergoing surgery for other reasons can result in lethal hypertension or arrhythmias.

**Breakout Point**

- Paroxysmal attacks of sweating, anxiety, headache, tremor, chest pain
- Paroxysmal hypertension, especially with surgery or pregnancy
- Diagnosis is made by increased 24-hour urine metanephrines

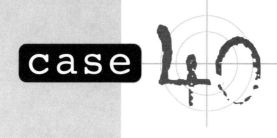

case 40

| | |
|---|---|
| **ID/CC** | A **27-year-old woman** presents with **amenorrhea** and infertility for the past year. |
| **HPI** | She reports decreased libido. She recently noticed **galactorrhea**. She denies **headaches** or **vision changes**. She takes no medications. |
| **PE** | VS: normal. PE: **bilateral nipple discharge;** no virilizing signs; normal visual fields. |
| **Labs** | Chem 7: normal BUN and creatinine. Serum HCG: negative. TSH: normal. **Serum prolactin: high.** |
| **Imaging** | **MRI with gadolinium:** small mass in anterior lobe of pituitary. |

# case 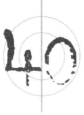 40

## Prolactinoma

**Pathogenesis**

**Prolactinomas** are benign neoplasms of the pituitary gland. Normally, prolactin stimulates lactation. Elevated levels of prolactin, however, cause **inhibition of gonadotropin-releasing hormone (GnRH)**, which causes inhibition of luteinizing hormone (LH). Symptoms tend to correlate with the level of prolactin and thus with the size of the tumor. The majority of young women tend to present early with microadenomas. Postmenopausal women and men tend to present late with adenoma size-related symptoms. Because postmenopausal women are functionally hypogonad, their adenomas may only be recognized once they have grown to cause neurologic symptoms. Men typically present late with hypogonadism, decreased libido, impotence, infertility, gynecomastia, or rarely galactorrhea. Of note, patients with **chronic renal insufficiency** have decreased prolactin clearance. **Dopamine receptor (D2) antagonists such as antipsychotics** decrease dopamine levels and thus can exacerbate hyperprolactinemia.

**Epidemiology**

Forty percent of all pituitary tumors are prolactin-secreting tumors; this is the most common hormone-secreting tumor of the pituitary.

**Management**

Treatment should include a dopamine agonist, such as **bromocriptine** or cabergoline. Indications to treat are hypogonadism or neurologic symptoms (current or impending). Ninety-five percent of untreated microadenomas do not change in size over 4 to 6 years. Bromocriptine is preferred for restoring fertility to female patients. **Transsphenoidal surgery** is considered for patients who have failed dopamine agonist therapy, or in women with large microadenomas who wish to become pregnant. Other women may opt for oral contraceptive therapy and yearly monitoring with prolactin levels. Prolactin levels are increased during pregnancy or physical or psychological stress; thus it is recommended to **check for possible pregnancy** prior to imaging. Any patient with a mass that extends beyond the sella should undergo a visual exam and anterior pituitary function testing.

**Complications**

Neurologic symptoms (headache or vision loss) can occur from enlarging adenoma. Osteopenia for both sexes may occur after long-standing hyperprolactinemia.

**Breakout Point**

- ↑Prolactin and ↓GnRH leads to hypogonadism
- Presents with amenorrhea, galactorrhea, infertility, decreased libido
- Bitemporal hemianopsia from optic chiasm compression
- Treated with bromocriptine

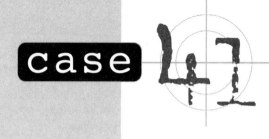
# case 47

| | |
|---|---|
| **ID/CC** | An **81-year-old woman** presents with **altered mental status, irritability,** and **confusion** over the past day. |
| **HPI** | Her family notes that she has had occasional episodes of previously unreported **intermittent hemoptysis** and chest pain over the past 3 months. She has **smoked** 2 packs of cigarettes per day for 60 years. |
| **PE** | VS: **normal BP.** PE: disoriented; lung, cardiac, and abdominal exams normal; **no edema present.** |
| **Labs** | CBC: normal. Lytes: **hyponatremia** (128 mEq/L). **Low serum osmolality** (<280 mOsm/kg); **elevated urine sodium** (>20 mmol/L); **concentrated urine** (increased urine osmolality); **detectable plasma ADH** (normally unmeasurable); cytology of sputum demonstrates malignant cells consistent with **small cell carcinoma.** |
| **Imaging** | CXR: hilar masses with mediastinal widening. |

case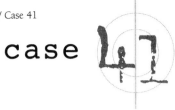

## Syndrome of Inappropriate Secretion of Antidiuretic Hormone (SIADH)

Pathogenesis

SIADH characteristically produces dilutional hyponatremia without edema. ADH is normally released from the posterior pituitary in response to serum osmolality or volume changes. ADH release is regulated by the CNS and by baroreceptors in the chest; thus, intrinsic causes of SIADH stem from disorders of the CNS and lungs. ADH may be ectopically produced from neoplasms (**small-cell lung carcinoma,** duodenal carcinoma, pancreatic carcinoma), from tuberculous lung parenchyma, following **intracranial lesions** (meningitis, trauma, encephalitis, SAH), or from drug-induced stimulation of ADH release (vincristine, chlorpropamide, carbamazepine) or potentiation of ADH effects (chlorpropamide, NSAIDs).

Management

Correct hyponatremia with **water restriction,** sodium replacement, and loop diuretics. Correct serum sodium to a normal range slowly in order to prevent the development of **central pontine myelinolysis.** Restrict fluid intake or administer saline depending on the patient's volume status. Causes of SIADH should be identified and corrected. Demeclocycline is the most potent inhibitor of ADH action and may be useful for chronic SIADH (untreatable malignancy or CNS disease).

Complications

Complications include confusion, seizures, or coma. Prognosis depends on the primary etiology.

Breakout Point

- Rapid correction of serum sodium can result in central pontine myelinolysis
- ADH is ectopically produced by small-cell carcinoma of the lung
- ADH can be produced following intracranial lesions

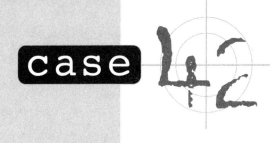

# case 42

**ID/CC** A **45-year-old woman** complains of **palpitations**.

**HPI** She also reports **fatigue** (due to anemia), **dysphagia** (due to oropharyngeal candidiasis secondary to neutropenia), and **easy bruising** and **epistaxis** (due to thrombocytopenia). She was recently hospitalized with **pneumonia**.

**PE** VS: **fever** (38.7°C); mild tachycardia (HR 105). PE: **pallor**; numerous bruises; **petechial hemorrhages** on tonsils and skin; **gum hypertrophy**; white oropharyngeal plaques; axillary **lymphadenopathy**; **sternal tenderness; hepatosplenomegaly**.

**Labs** CBC/PBS: **anemia** (Hb 9); **low platelet count** (40,000); **leukopenia** (2,000); **circulating blasts with Auer rods** (Figure 42-2). Elevated uric acid and LDH. UA: hyperuricosuria (secondary to increased cell turnover). **Bone marrow biopsy** reveals **increased proportion of blast cells** (>20%) with prominent **staining with peroxidase and Sudan black** as well as staining for CD33 and CD13 cytogenetic testing reveals 15:17 translocation.

**Imaging** CXR: no mediastinal mass (presence of mediastinal mass would suggest T-cell ALL).

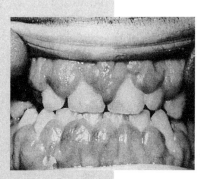

**Figure 42-1.** Gum hypertrophy.

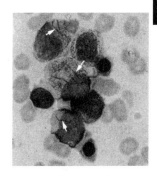

**Figure 42-2.** Circulating blasts with Auer rods (*arrows*).

83

case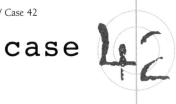

## Acute Myelogenous Leukemia (AML)

**Pathogenesis**

Acute myelogenous leukemia (AML) arises most commonly as a result of **clonal proliferation** of multipotential precursors of granulocytes, macrophages, erythrocytes, and megakaryocytes. The most common risk factor is the **presence of antecedent hematologic disorders** such as myelodysplastic syndrome (most common), aplastic anemia, myelofibrosis, paroxysmal nocturnal hemoglobinuria, and polycythemia vera. Other etiologic factors include **heredity** (chromosome aneuploidy syndromes such as Down and Klinefelter syndromes or diseases with excessive chromosome fragility such as Fanconi anemia or Bloom syndrome), **radiation, chemical exposure** (e.g., benzene), and **antineoplastic drugs** (e.g., alkylating agents). Several subtypes of AML have been attributed to translocations that lead to the production of oncogenic proteins: (15;17) in M3. Replacement of normal marrow with leukemic marrow leads to pancytopenia and to the sequelae of the disease.

**Epidemiology**

Seen more commonly in individuals **older than 60 years** and in patients with **chronic myeloproliferative disorders and myelodysplastic syndromes.** APL subtype is seen more commonly in younger patients (median age 40).

**Management**

Use of **ATRA (all-*trans*-retinoic acid)** improves the outcome in M3 AML (as in this case). Remission may be achieved using induction **chemotherapy** followed by intensive postremission chemotherapy or **bone marrow transplant** (allogeneic or autologous). Recurrences are effectively treated only with bone marrow transplant.

**Complications**

Patients often develop substantial **local and disseminated infections,** bleeding complications (DIC, GI bleeding), urate nephropathy, and cerebral leukostasis. Those receiving bone marrow transplants may develop **graft-versus-host disease.** Relapse may occur.

**Breakout Point**

- Translocation in AML M3 subtype is t(15;17)
- Auer rod is pathognomonic
- PML-RARalpha fusion protein
- Treated with all-*trans* retinoic acid
- DIC in M3 AML can cause widespread bleeding

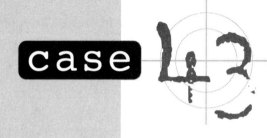

# case 43

**ID/CC**  A **29-year-old woman** presents to the clinic complaining of **persistent fatigue and weakness.**

**HPI**  She states that she has **heavy menstrual bleeding** (MENORRHAGIA) and frequent **bleeding between periods** (METRORRHAGIA). She adds that she has **brittle nails** and frequently **eats ice** (PICA).

**PE**  VS: normal. PE: **pallor;** no scleral icterus; moist mucous membranes; **atrophic tongue;** 2-sec capillary refill; regular rate and rhythm.

**Labs**  CBC: hypochromic, microcytic RBCs; **low hemoglobin** (9 g/dL) **and hematocrit** (28%); elevated RDW; low MCV and MCHC. **Serum iron depressed; ferritin low; TIBC elevated.**

**Imaging**  None.

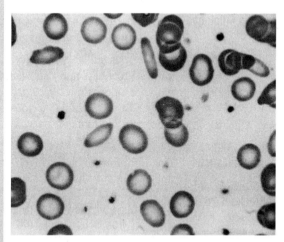

**Figure 43-1.** Hypochromic, microcytic RBCs.

HEME/ONC

85

# case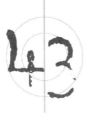

## Anemia—Iron Deficiency

**Pathogenesis**

Iron is absorbed preferentially in the duodenum and proximal jejunum, so conditions that bypass or otherwise decrease absorption may lead to anemia. Iron deficiency may also develop in conditions where blood is lost through the **GI** (peptic ulcer, gastritis, hemorrhoids, angiodysplasia, parasites, and malignancy) **or GU tract, in menstruation,** and in conditions of **increased iron demand such as pregnancy or adolescence.** Depleted iron stores result in hemoglobin-deficient cells and consequent hypochromia and microcytosis. Iron-deficiency anemia is defined by low serum iron (although recent intake of iron can increase serum iron), low ferritin (storage form of iron in the bone marrow), and high TIBC (total iron-binding capacity).

**Epidemiology**

Iron deficiency is the **most common form of anemia in the United States,** appearing in **20% of U.S. women.**

**Management**

Oral ferrous sulfate will yield a brisk reticulocytosis within 3 to 4 days and a substantial increase in hemoglobin in approximately 10 days. In patients who are unable to tolerate oral ferrous sulfate, oral ferrous gluconate and fumarate as well as a parenteral formulation are available.

**Complications**

Complications include high-output cardiac failure and Plummer–Vinson syndrome.

**Breakout Point**

- Microcytic (low MCV), hypochromic (low MCHC) ↓ iron, ↓ ferritin, ↑ TIBC
- Associated with pica and restless leg syndrome

Plummer Vincent Syndrome =
1) Iron deficiency anemia
2) esophageal web
3) atrophic glossitis

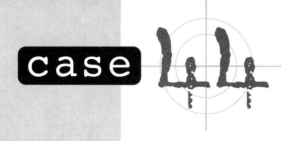

| | |
|---|---|
| ID/CC | A **50-year-old vegan woman** presents with **pallor** and **fatigue**. |
| HPI | She also reports **spastic weakness** of both legs and **anesthesia** progressing proximally from her distal extremities (GLOVE-AND-STOCKING DISTRIBUTION). |
| PE | VS: normal. PE: pallor; mild icterus; **beefy-red tongue** (GLOSSITIS); **loss of balance, vibratory, and position sense** in both lower extremities; decreased sensation in distal extremities; spastic weakness of lower extremities with absent DTRs; **slapping gait** (proprioceptive loss); Babinski present bilaterally; hepatosplenomegaly. |
| Labs | CBC/PBS: **decreased hemoglobin; high MCV** (MACRO-CYTIC ANEMIA); mild leukopenia (4,000) with **hypersegmented neutrophils** (Figure 44-1); thrombocytopenia. Low serum cobalamin; achlorhydria (no hydrochloric acid in gastric juice); Schilling test consistent with **intrinsic factor deficiency;** antibodies against parietal cells and intrinsic factor demonstrated; homocystinemia; hypermethioninemia; bone marrow smear reveals marked erythroid hyperplasia. UA: homocystinuria. |
| Imaging | None. |

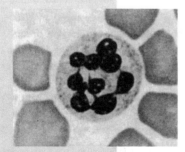

**Figure 44-1.** Hypersegmented neutrophil.

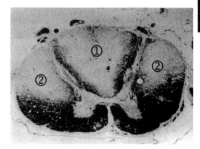

**Figure 44-2.** Subacute combined degeneration of the spinal cord with characteristic involvement of posterior (1) and lateral (2) tracts, and progressive peripheral neuropathy.

HEME/ONC

87

# case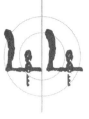

## Anemia—Vitamin B$_{12}$ Deficiency

**Pathogenesis**

The absorption of vitamin B$_{12}$ (also known as cobalamin) requires (1) adequate dietary intake (**vitamin B$_{12}$ is found only in animal products** such as meat, liver, fish, eggs, and milk), (2) production of **intrinsic factor** by the gastric antrum, and (3) uptake of the intrinsic factor–vitamin complex by the terminal ileum. The most common cause is **pernicious anemia** or atrophic gastritis results in decreased intrinsic factor production with subsequent malabsorption of vitamin B$_{12}$. The same effect results from partial or total **gastrectomy**. Diseases affecting the **terminal ileum** (e.g., Crohn disease and intestinal lymphoma) can prevent the uptake of the intrinsic factor–vitamin B$_{12}$ complex. **Blind-loop syndrome** results in bacterial overgrowth within the intestine, resulting in consumption of vitamin B$_{12}$ before uptake can occur. In severe cases of prolonged malnutrition or **strict vegan diet**, vitamin B$_{12}$ deficiency may occur because of decreased intake. Generally, nutritional deficiency is a rare cause of vitamin B$_{12}$ deficiency because of large liver stores (2 to 4 mg) that are sufficient for years to decades. A rare cause is infection with the fish tapeworm, *Diphyllobothrium latum,* which has a high affinity for vitamin B$_{12}$. The Schilling test is designed to identify the cause of vitamin B$_{12}$ deficiency, but is rarely used.

**Epidemiology**

More common among patients with chronic malnutrition and among those with minimal or no meat consumption (vegans).

**Management**

**Regular IM vitamin B$_{12}$** supplementation.

**Complications**

Macrocytic, megaloblastic anemia, glossitis, confusion, depression, psychosis ("megaloblastic madness"), decreased phagocyte and PMN response, subacute combined degeneration of the spinal cord with characteristic involvement of posterior and lateral tracts, and progressive peripheral neuropathy (Figure 44-2).

**Breakout Point**

- Most common cause—pernicious anemia
- Macrocytic, megaloblastic anemia
- Hypersegmented neutrophils
- Subacute combined degeneration of the spinal cord

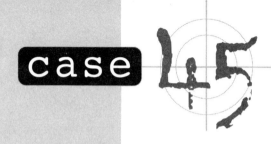

**case 45**

| | |
|---|---|
| **ID/CC** | A **53-year-old woman** presents for a **routine physical.** |
| **HPI** | It has been **5 years since she was last seen by a physician.** She has a history of a left breast lump at her last physical examination; needle biopsy of the lump revealed fibrocystic breast disease. |
| **PE** | VS: normal. PE: notable for slight **focal pitted skin (peau d'orange)** in the inferior aspect of the **right breast skin;** breast exam reveals a small **palpable mass** subjacent to the pitted skin. |
| **Labs** | CBC/Lytes: normal. |
| **Imaging** | Mammography: **stellate 1-cm mass in the right breast** with overlying skin thickening. The left breast shows benign-appearing calcifications, changes consistent with fibrocystic breast disease, and a clip marking the prior biopsy site. |
| **Histology** | A core needle biopsy of the mass reveals **well-differentiated** (grade I) **infiltrating ductal carcinoma.** Immunohistochemical stains (antibodies that stain specific antigens on cells) reveal the tumor cells to be positive for estrogen receptor (ER), progesterone receptor (PR), and for ErbB2 (HER2/neu). |

HEME/ONC

# case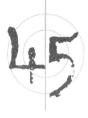

## Breast Cancer

**Pathogenesis**

The precursor lesion of invasive ductal breast cancer is **ductal carcinoma in situ** (DCIS). Risk factors include **family history (first-degree relative with breast cancer), age, early menarche/late menopause, late age at first delivery, and nulliparity.** Lobular carcinoma in situ (LCIS) is also a risk factor. Unlike DCIS, LCIS is not considered a precursor lesion. Less commonly, those with genetic mutations involving **BRCA1 or BRCA2** (both of which are tumor suppressor genes) have roughly a 60% chance of developing breast cancer by age 50.

**Epidemiology**

In the United States, breast cancer is the most common cancer in women and the second most common cause of cancer-related deaths in women. **Infiltrating ductal carcinoma,** the most common subtype, accounts for more than 70% of all cases. Other common subtypes include lobular and ductal with lobular features accounting for roughly 16.

**Management**

Management and prognosis are dictated by the **cancer grade and subtype, stage, and ER/PR/HER2/neu status** at time of diagnosis. Early-stage cancers (stage I and II) can be treated conservatively with **lumpectomy and radiation,** or with **modified radical mastectomy** with or without radiation. Both procedures are equivalent in survival rates. Sentinel lymph node sampling is also performed. Treatment modalities for stage III and IV cancers may include chemotherapy, radiation, hormonal, and surgical therapy. Expression of ER and PR are predictors of good prognosis and response to hormonal therapy. Expression of HER2/neu avails treatment with **trastuzumab (Herceptin),** a monoclonal antibody against ErbB2. Imaging should be obtained to check for metastasis.

**Complications**

Recurrence, seroma, and lymphedema.

**Breakout Point**

- Screening: yearly mammograms starting at age 40 and earlier in those with risk factors
- Risk factors: age, positive family history, early menarche/late menopause, late age at first delivery, nulliparity

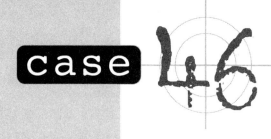

case 46

ID/CC  A **14-year-old boy** is brought to the ER because of **abdominal pain** and **distention, inability to evacuate and pass flatus per rectum,** nausea, and **vomiting** (intestinal obstruction).

HPI  He is a healthy boy who is fully immunized and has not traveled outside the United States.

PE  VS: slight fever (38.3°C); tachycardia (HR 102); tachypnea (RR 22); normal BP. PE: dehydration; no jaundice; pallor; neck supple with no lymphadenopathy; **abdomen distended, tympanitic,** and tender; bowel sounds increased; no peritoneal signs; no masses; no hepatosplenomegaly; laparotomy reveals an **ileal mass** that produced an intussusception.

Labs  CBC: normocytic anemia; mild leukocytosis; no neutrophilia. **Elevated LDH;** tumor aspirate sent for intraoperative cytology reveals Burkitt lymphoma cells (basophilic, nongranular nuclei; high mitotic index; 2 to 5 nucleoli; eccentric, thin cytoplasm) on Romanowsky stain (Wright or Giemsa); histopathology of mass reveals **"starry sky" pattern.**

Imaging  None.

case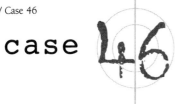

## Burkitt Lymphoma

**Pathogenesis**

Burkitt lymphoma is a high-grade, undifferentiated B-lymphocyte **lymphoblastic lymphoma** that has two major clinical presentations. The **African type** is endemic, is associated with EBV infection, and presents as a jaw or abdominal tumor that may spread to the bone marrow. The **American** type is sporadic and has an abdominal presentation that includes ascites along with skin, bone, and peripheral node involvement. Most patients carry a translocation of the **c-myc** oncogene t(8; 14). **Predisposing** factors include **EBV** (African type), **malaria** (mitogenic for B lymphocytes; causes defective cellular immunity), or periodontal infections. also t(8,2) or t(8,22)

**Epidemiology**

A **pediatric** disease with **a mean age of onset of 7** that occurs **more often in males.** It is the most common malignant pediatric tumor in Africa and the most rapidly growing malignant tumor in humans (may double in size in 24 hours).

**Management**

Most treatment regimens include brief high-dose combination chemotherapy with CNS prophylaxis. Chemotherapy can cause **tumor lysis syndrome,** which presents with joint pains, hyperkalemia, hyperphosphatemia, hypocalcemia, and hyperuricemia. Recurrences arise within the first 6 months, usually in the CNS.

**Complications**

Metastatic and recurrent disease, bleeding, and infection.

**Breakout Point**

- High-grade B-cell neoplasm
- Associated with EBV
- "Starry-sky" pattern on histopathology
- Higher incidence in Africans than Americans

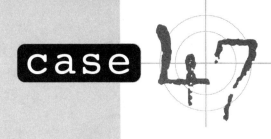

# case 47

| | |
|---|---|
| **ID/CC** | A **66-year-old man** presents for a routine physical. |
| **HPI** | The patient has **no complaints**. |
| **PE** | PE: pallor, **palpable axillary lymph nodes;** splenomegaly; hepatomegaly. |
| **Labs** | CBC/PBS: **anemia; thrombocytopenia; lymphocytosis** (>15,000); reduced serum immunoglobulins; **bone marrow biopsy reveals diffuse infiltration by mature lymphocytes;** lymphocyte marker analysis reveals CD19, CD20, CD21, and CD24 (B-CELL ANTIGENS). |
| **Imaging** | Peripheral smear: small, mature lymphocytes and smudge cells (Figure 47-1). |

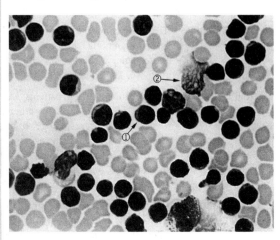

**Figure 47-1. Mature,** slightly smaller lymphocytes (*1*) and **smudge cells** (*2*).

HEME/ONC

case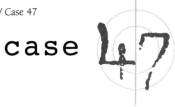

## Chronic Lymphocytic Leukemia (CLL)

**Pathogenesis**

Chronic lymphocytic leukemia (CLL) is a neoplasm that usually arises from clonal proliferation of activated **B-cells** (>95%). Its etiology is unknown, but several chromosomal abnormalities, including deletion of 13q and trisomy 12, have been identified. Chromosomal abnormalities are associated with shortened survival. Patients with CLL are staged on the basis of nodal involvement and the presence of anemia or thrombocytopenia. In the Binet staging classification, **stage A** is lymphocytosis with <3 lymph node groups; **stage B** includes involvement of >3 lymph node groups; and **stage C** is assigned in the presence of anemia or thrombocytopenia, which may be due to bone marrow compromise, spleen involvement, or an autoimmune cause.

**Epidemiology**

The **most common form of adult leukemia** in the United States, accounting for 25% to 40% of all cases and increasing in frequency with age (90% of cases occur in patients older than 50). The disease is uncommon in Asian countries.

**Management**

Start treatment when patients are symptomatic. Stage A patients do not receive chemotherapy given that their survival is >10 years; stage B and C patients require **chemotherapy** (alkylating agents, fludarabine, pentostatin, cladribine). **Glucocorticoids** or splenectomy can be useful in cases of Coombs-positive hemolytic anemia, immune thrombocytopenia, and pancytopenia.

**Complications**

CLL may transform into a **prolymphocytic leukemia** or a **high-grade lymphoma.** Patients are also susceptible to infections (due to hypogammaglobulinemia) such as pneumococcal pneumonia and shingles as well as to hematologic derangements such as anemia, thrombocytopenia, and neutropenia.

**Breakout Point**

- Asymptomatic, elderly patients
- Mature lymphocytosis and smudge cells
- Splenomegaly is common

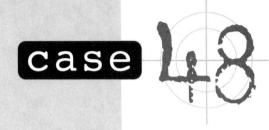

**ID/CC**  A **46-year-old man** complains of **easy fatigability** and **weakness**.

**HPI**  He acknowledges recent **weight loss, anorexia, abdominal fullness** (due to massive splenomegaly), and **night sweats**.

**PE**  VS: **low-grade fever** (38.5°C). PE: pallor; no lymphadenopathy; **splenomegaly** palpable 10 cm below costal margin; hepatomegaly.

**Labs**  CBC/PBS: **elevated WBC** (>100,000); decreased hemoglobin (9); thrombocytosis; **many mature neutrophils, promyelocytes, metamyelocytes, and myelocytes** (<10% myeloblasts). Serum $B_{12}$ and uric acid elevated; decreased leukocyte alkaline phosphatase; **bone marrow biopsy reveals hypercellularity with elevated myeloid-to-erythroid ratio** (10:1).

**Imaging**  See Figure 48-1.

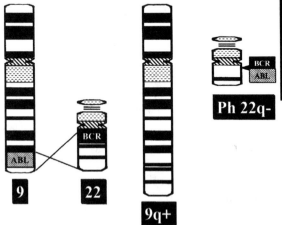

**Figure 48-1. Translocation** (9:22) (BCR-ABL FUSION GENE OR PHILADELPHIA CHROMOSOME).

case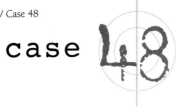

## Chronic Myelogenous Leukemia (CML)

**Pathogenesis**

Chronic myelogenous leukemia (CML) is a **myeloproliferative disease** that is characterized by clonal expansion of neoplastic pluripotent stem cells. In >90% of cases, the disease arises following the formation of the **bcr-abl fusion gene**, which produces an overexpressing tyrosine kinase.

**Epidemiology**

Occurs most commonly in the fourth to fifth decades with a **slight male predominance** and accounts for 15% to 20% of all leukemia cases. Survivors of the atomic bombs in Japan developed CML at an increased, dose-dependent rate, with most cases arising 5 to 12 years after exposure. Median survival is approximately 3 to 4 years.

**Management**

For patients who can tolerate transplant and who have donors, **allogenic bone marrow transplant** often offers the best hope for cure. **Imatinib mesylate (Gleevec)**, which acts by directly inhibiting the tyrosine kinase activity produced by the bcr-abl fusion gene, is the agent of choice. CML has a biphasic or triphasic clinical course. The **chronic phase** behaves as a benign neoplasm and can be managed with chemotherapy or immunotherapy. Patients in the chronic phase are frequently given **hydroxyurea** to minimize the leukemic cell burden. CML progresses to a **blastic phase** that resembles acute leukemia with or without an intervening **accelerated phase**.

**Complications**

Hyperviscosity and/or thrombocytosis; predisposition to cerebrovascular accidents, neuropathies, and splenic infarcts.

**Breakout Point**

- Philadelphia chromosome: t(9;22)
- bcr-abl fusion protein causes tyrosine kinase overactivity
- Blast crisis in late phase looks like acute leukemia

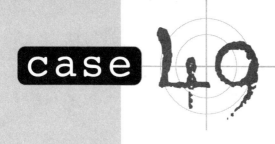

case 49

| | |
|---|---|
| **ID/CC** | A **29-year-old woman** complains of left **lower extremity pain and swelling.** |
| **HPI** | Her symptoms started 2 days after returning home from vacation. She first noticed a dull ache in the back of her calf, which progressed to swelling, tenderness, and discoloration from her ankle to her knee. |
| **PE** | VSS. PE: nonpitting edema in left lower extremity, with diffuse erythema and tenderness; no palpable cord but **Homan sign** (pain in the calf with passive dorsiflexion of the foot) is present. |
| **Labs** | CBC, PT, PTT, INR within normal limits; **D-dimer elevated.** |
| **Imaging** | **US lower extremity:** occlusive thrombus in deep vein of left calf. |

# case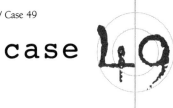

## Deep Vein Thrombosis

**Pathogenesis**

A deep venous thrombosis (DVT) is composed of red blood cells, fibrin, and platelets. DVTs occur as a result of the **Virchow triad:** vessel wall injury, coagulopathy, and venous stasis. Exposure of subendothelial collagen and tissue factor causes platelet adhesion and activation of the extrinsic coagulation cascade. The thrombus expands if the balance of procoagulants and anticoagulants favors further thrombus formation.

**Epidemiology**

50% of DVTs and PEs are asymptomatic and undetected. Proximal DVTs (from the popliteal vein to the distal IVC) are more likely to cause pulmonary embolus. Risk factors that lead to DVT formation include increased **age, estrogen exposure (postpartum, OCP, hormone replacement therapy),** bed rest, **surgery, immobility** (long plane or car trips), and **malignancy.**

**Management**

DVT is treated by **anticoagulation,** starting with either unfractionated heparin or low-molecular-weight heparin (lovenox) as a bridge to a therapeutic INR (international normalized ratio) on warfarin (usually in a range of 2.0 to 3.0). The length of treatment depends on the clinical scenario, but ranges from 6 to 12 months. Only high-risk patients need lifelong anticoagulation. If the patient has no known risk factors for DVT, a hypercoagulable workup and age-appropriate cancer screening should be performed.

**Complications**

Propagation of a thrombus can lead to total venous obstruction and pulmonary emboli (PE). Other complications include varicose veins, chronic venous insufficiency, and bleeding (while anticoagulated).

**Breakout Point**

- Ultrasound of lower extremity for diagnosis
- Unclear etiology of DVT leads to suspicion for hypercoagulability/malignancy
- Factor V Leiden is the most common inherited cause

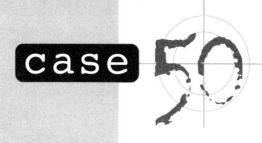

# case 50

**ID/CC** A 42-year-old woman hospitalized in the ICU for *E. coli* **sepsis** begins to display extensive skin and mucous membrane **bleeding**.

**HPI** She is being treated with IV antibiotics and is on pressor therapy.

**PE** VS: tachycardia (HR 129); hypotension (BP 66/42); breathing with assisted ventilation. PE: unresponsive; multiple **diffuse petechiae** and hematomas; **bleeding from IV and pulmonary artery catheter sites.**

**Labs** CBC: thrombocytopenia. PBS: schistocytes. Prolonged PT/PTT; low fibrinogen; low clotting factors; elevated fibrin degradation products; elevated D-dimer.

**Imaging** None.

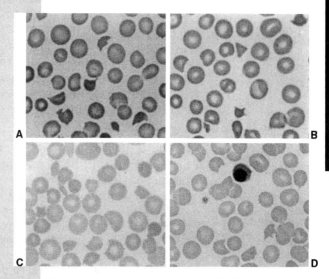

**Figure 50-1.** Schistocytes in patients with TTP **(A)**, DIC **(B)**, aortic valve replacement **(C)**, and HUS **(D)**.

HEME/ONC

# case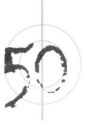

## Disseminated Intravascular Coagulation (DIC)

**Pathogenesis**

Disseminated intravascular coagulation (DIC) is characterized by a generalized activation of the coagulation system that may present with varying degrees of severity. It is most frequently associated with **sepsis, burns, obstetric complications (amniotic fluid embolism, intrauterine fetal death, septic abortion), metastatic malignancy, massive trauma,** and organ destruction (severe **pancreatitis**). A potent thrombogenic stimulus causes thrombosis production throughout the microvasculature, followed by a hemorrhagic phase marked by procoagulant factor consumption and secondary fibrinolysis.

**Management**

**Correct the underlying disorder** (e.g., infection). Control bleeding or thrombosis. Administer **fresh frozen plasma** to replace depleted clotting factors, blood and platelet concentrates to correct thrombocytopenia, and low-dose **IV heparin** in cases of thrombosis. Treat chronic DIC with periodic plasma and platelet replacement. DIC is unresponsive to warfarin; heparin may be administered by periodic injection or continuous infusion.

**Complications**

Complications include death, uncontrollable hemorrhage, ARDS, thrombosis of vessels, and pregangrenous changes in the digits, nose, and genitalia. Microinfarctions and thrombi can also be found in the heart, liver, kidneys, and brain.

**Breakout Point**

- Signifies a serious underlying disorder
- Consumptive coagulopathy of both bleeding and thrombosis
- ↑PT, ↑PTT, ↓fibrinogen, ↑fibrin degradation (split) products

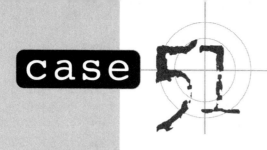

case 51

**ID/CC**     An **18-year-old man** presents with an acutely **painful** and **swollen knee.**

**HPI**     He fell while playing basketball this morning. Several hours later he developed a warm sensation in his right knee followed by severe pain and swelling. He reports a history of **easy bruising** and **bleeding** since childhood. He has never had any dental or surgical procedures. Family history is significant for a maternal grandfather who died at age 30 from **delayed postoperative bleeding complications.**

**PE**     VS: normal. PE: right knee joint is warm, markedly swollen, with painful limited range of motion; no erythema; multiple **large ecchymoses** on extremities.

**Labs**     CBC: mild anemia; PT normal; **aPTT prolonged**; bleeding time normal; **factor VIII activity decreased.**

**Imaging**     X-ray, knee: effusion and soft-tissue swelling.

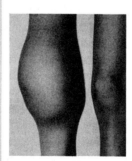

**Figure 51-1.** Cross knee effusion.

HEME/ONC

# case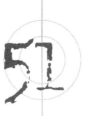

## Hemophilia A

**Pathogenesis**

Hemophilia A is an **X-linked recessive** disorder caused by deficiency or impaired function of coagulation **factor VIII** (FVIII). Clinical severity correlates with level of the FVIII activity. Bleeding history is characterized by **spontaneous** and/or **delayed posttraumatic or postoperative bleeding into deep tissues, such as joints (hemarthrosis) and muscles.** (This pattern is different from the bleeding pattern that would suggest platelet dysfunction; petechiae and superficial mucocutaneous bleeding are typically absent.)

**Epidemiology**

Incidence of hemophilia A is about 1 per 10,000 live male births. Males express the disease and females are carriers (X-linked recessive inheritance). Family history may be "hidden" for many generations if no male children are born.

**Management**

**Recombinant factor VIII** is the mainstay of therapy. Recombinant factor VIIa (NovoSeven) may be used for those who develop FVIII inhibitor (alloantibodies to exogenous FVIII). In addition, desmopressin and antifibrinolytic therapy can also be used. Counsel patients regarding physical activity restrictions and avoidance of aspirin. Management of chronic complications, such as hemarthroses and transfusion-associated viral infections, requires referral to specialists.

**Complications**

Internal hemorrhage may cause airway obstruction, compartment syndrome, damage to internal organs (chronic arthropathy, neuropathy). Intracranial hemorrhage is associated with high mortality. Blood-borne viral infections (HIV, hepatitis) are common among patients who received transfusion products before the mid–1980s.

**Breakout Point**

- X-linked recessive (only males are affected; father cannot transmit the disease to sons, but all his daughters will be carriers)
- Five Hs: **H**emarthrosis, **H**ematomas, **H**ematochezia, **H**ematuria, and **H**ead hemorrhage

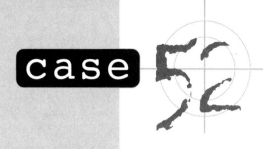

**ID/CC**    A **29-year-old man** presents complaining of **easy fatigability and lethargy.**

**HPI**    The patient states that he was diagnosed with **gallstones** several years ago and adds that his **mother had a splenectomy** while in her 20s.

**PE**    VS: normal. PE: **jaundice; scleral icterus**; abdomen soft, nontender, and nondistended; **splenomegaly**.

**Labs**    CBC: normal WBC; **decreased hemoglobin (9.5 g/dL) and hematocrit (28%); slightly decreased MCV; elevated MCHC**. PBS: **anisocytosis with numerous spherocytes; reticulocytosis**. LFTs: **unconjugated bilirubin elevated. Osmotic fragility test positive;** Coombs test negative.

**Imaging**    None.

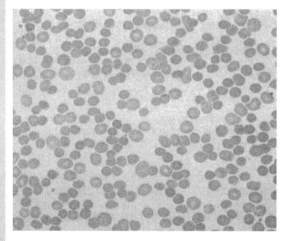

**Figure 52-1.** Anisocytosis with numerous spherocytes; reticulocytosis.

HEME/ONC

# case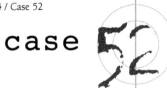

## Hereditary Spherocytosis

| | |
|---|---|
| **Pathogenesis** | Hereditary spherocytosis (HS) is an **autosomal-dominant** disorder characterized by cytoskeletal defects in the RBC membrane, yielding RBCs that are spheroidal, more rigid than normal, fragile, and at risk for splenic sequestration and lysis. The **most common defect occurs in spectrin**, a cytoskeletal element that ordinarily acts as a strut to support the RBC membrane and maintain its biconcave disk shape. Spectrin deficiency leads to a decrease in RBC surface area. Infection, particularly with parvovirus B19, may precipitate decompensation and aplastic crisis. |
| **Epidemiology** | HS is often diagnosed during childhood, although milder cases may be discovered in adult life. It is the most common hereditary hemolytic anemia among people of Northern European descent. |
| **Management** | RBC survival is dramatically enhanced with **splenectomy** despite the persistence of the cytoskeletal abnormality. Do not schedule splenectomy until after 4 years of age because of the risk of severe infection. Administer **polyvalent pneumococcal vaccine** prior to surgery. Give folic acid and iron supplementation as needed. |
| **Complications** | Chronic leg ulcers, gallstones, and folate deficiency. |
| **Breakout Point** | • Increased MCHC<br>• Abnormal osmotic fragility test<br>• Spectrin deficiency<br>• Autosomal dominant |

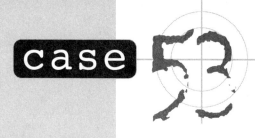

# case 53

**ID/CC**  A **35-year-old man** has been troubled by **fever, weight loss,** and drenching **night sweats** for the past several weeks.

**HPI**  He has no significant medical history. He reports occasional cough and shortness of breath during this period (hilar adenopathy).

**PE**  VS: fever (38.9°C). PE: **nontender cervical lymphadenopathy; hepatosplenomegaly.**

**Labs**  CBC: anemia; leukocytosis. Elevated ESR. LFTs: elevated serum alkaline phosphatase; elevated LDH. Lymph node biopsy reveals **binucleate giant cell** with eosinophilic inclusion-like nucleoli (REED–STERNBERG CELL).

**Imaging**  CXR, PA: widespread enlargement of hilar and mediastinal lymph nodes.

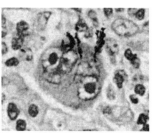

**Figure 53-2.** Lymph node biopsy reveals **binucleate giant cell** with eosinophilic inclusion-like nucleoli (REED–STERNBERG CELL).

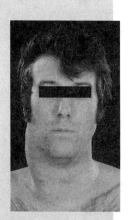

**Figure 53-1.** Nontender cervical lymphadenopathy.

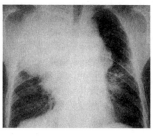

**Figure 53-3.** CXR, PA. Widespread enlargement of hilar and mediastinal lymph nodes.

HEME/ONC

case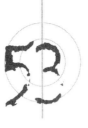

## Hodgkin Lymphoma

**Pathogenesis**

The etiology of Hodgkin lymphoma is unknown, although all forms are characterized by the presence of the Reed–Sternberg (RS) cell, a large cell with bilobate nucleoli. Hodgkin lymphoma is categorized in four forms: (1) **lymphocytic predominance,** which is the least common form, carries the best prognosis, and is characterized by a predominance of lymphocytic cells compared with RS cells; (2) **mixed cellularity,** which is associated with a good prognosis; (3) **lymphocytic depletion,** which carries the worst prognosis and is characterized by a proliferation of RS cells and a depletion of lymphocytes; and (4) **nodular sclerosis,** which is the most common form, carries a good prognosis and is characterized by nodular division of affected lymph nodes by fibrous bands and by the presence of lacunar cells.

**Epidemiology**

The incidence of Hodgkin lymphoma is **higher in men** (commonly occurring between 15 and 35 years of age, with another peak in those older than 50 years) than in women except for the nodular sclerosis form. EBV may be involved in the pathogenesis of Hodgkin disease.

**Management**

**Radiation** is indicated for focal disease (stage IA or IIA). Disseminated disease should be treated with aggressive **combination chemotherapy.** The treatment of choice appears to be doxorubicin (Adriamycin), bleomycin, vincristine, and dacarbazine (ABVD). A combination of therapies may be indicated for advanced disease.

**Complications**

Chemotherapeutic modalities used (ABVD) may be associated with a long-term risk of secondary leukemias and infertility. Mediastinal irradiation leads to paresthesias, sclerosis of coronary arteries (increased risk of MI), pulmonary fibrosis, pericardial effusions, and hypothyroidism.

**Breakout Point**

- Painless lymphadenopathy in the neck
- B symptoms: fever, weight loss, night sweats
- Types: lymphocyte predominance, nodular sclerosis, mixed cellularity, lymphocyte depletion

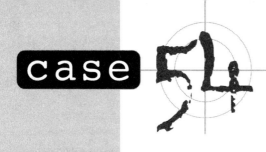

# case 54

**ID/CC** A **35-year-old woman** presents with a 7-month history of **easy bruising.**

**HPI** She notices bruising primarily over her extremities after bumping into furniture and other objects. She has also had occasional **gum bleeding** when brushing her teeth and episodes of **epistaxis.** She denies hematochezia, melena, menorrhagia, and hematuria. She denies recent viral illness and new medications.

**PE** VS: Normal. PE: scattered ecchymoses on upper and lower extremities; **petechial rash on bilateral lower extremities.**

**Labs** CBC: **platelet count 30 (very low).** PT, PTT, INR: normal.

**Imaging** None.

case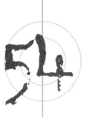

## Idiopathic Thrombocytopenic Purpura (ITP)

**Pathogenesis**
Immune (idiopathic) thrombocytopenic purpura (ITP) is a diagnosis of exclusion characterized by **autoimmune destruction of platelets**. ITP is mediated by IgG autoantibodies directed against platelets, causing their phagocytosis and **destruction in the reticuloendothelial system**. The decreased number of platelets results in mild bleeding manifestations including bruising, petechiae, purpura, and mucosal bleeding. Severe bleeding is rare.

**Epidemiology**
Acute ITP is a brief self-limited illness typically seen in children and young adults, and often related to a viral illness. Chronic ITP has a more insidious onset, with patients typically presenting after months of bruising and mild bleeding.

**Management**
Once a diagnosis of ITP has been made, treatment is initiated for those patients with moderate or severe thrombocytopenia. There is no absolute number of platelets below which treatment is recommended, but significant bleeding is seen more commonly at platelet counts <10,000/µL. **Corticosteroids** should be used as initial therapy. If severe thrombocytopenia persists or relapses, **intravenous immunoglobulin (IVIG), Rituximab (anti-CD20), and/or splenectomy** are available treatment options.

**Complications**
Intracranial hemorrhage is the most feared complication.

**Breakout Point**

- Antiplatelet antibodies
- Isolated thrombocytopenia
- Normal PT, PTT
- Treat with corticosteroids

■ TABLE 54-1 DIFFERENTIATION OF ACUTE AND CHRONIC ITP AT CLINICAL PRESENTATION

| Parameter | Acute ITP | Chronic ITP |
|---|---|---|
| Age (yr) | <10 | >10 |
| Sex | M = F | F > M |
| Onset of symptoms | Abrupt | Insidious |
| Viral prodome | Yes | No |
| Platelet count | <20 × 10⁹/L | 20–50 × 10⁹/L |
| Platelet-associated IgG | Markedly elevated | Modestly elevated |
| Family history of autoimmune disease | No | Occasionally |
| Other immunologic abnormalities | No | Occasionally |

IgG, Immunoglobin G.

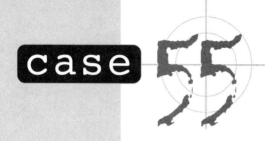

# case 55

| | |
|---|---|
| **ID/CC** | A **59-year-old African American man** seeks attention for **lower back pain**. |
| **HPI** | He also complains of **fatigue** and **rib tenderness**. |
| **PE** | VS: normal. PE: **pallor**; petechiae on buccal mucosa; **bone tenderness** on pressing ribs and spine; no hepatosplenomegaly; blanching and cyanosis of fingers, toes, tips of nose, and earlobes (RAYNAUD PHENOMENON). |
| **Labs** | CBC/PBS: normocytic **anemia** (Hb 8.0); **leukopenia**; rouleaux formation. **Markedly elevated ESR.** Hypercalcemia; hypogammaglobulinemia; increased serum total protein; serum protein electrophoresis shows a **monoclonal spike** (M protein) on beta- or gamma-globulin region (MONOCLONAL GAMMOPATHY); bone marrow shows replacement of normal marrow elements by plasma cells. UA: increased uric acid; phosphaturia; glucosuria; **Bence Jones proteinuria** (IgG light chains). |
| **Imaging** | XR, skull: punched-out (OSTEOLYTIC) lesions in the skull with generalized **osteoporosis** (bone scan is not useful; no uptake due to lack of osteoblastic component). |

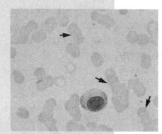

**Figure 55-1.** Rouleaux formations (*arrows*).

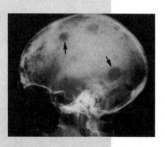

**Figure 55-3.** XR, skull. Punched-out (OSTEOLYTIC) lesions in the skull (arrows) with generalized **osteoporosis**.

**Figure 55-2.** Bone marrow shows replacement of normal marrow elements by plasma cells (*arrows*).

HEME/ONC

# case 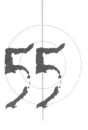 55

## Multiple Myeloma

**Pathogenesis**

Multiple myeloma is a primary **malignant proliferation of plasma cells in the bone marrow,** with resulting marrow failure and overproduction of immunoglobulin. Serum immunoelectrophoresis shows a **monoclonal elevation of one immunoglobulin** (detected by serum protein electrophoresis) with a reciprocal depression of the other classes of immunoglobulins. The bone pain and lesions result from tumor growth and from increased osteoclast activity (induced by cytokines produced by myeloma cells). Pneumonia and UTIs are common. Renal failure (25% of patients develop **myeloma kidney**) results from several factors, including hyperuricemia, hypercalcemia, infection, and the **excretion of light chains.**

**Epidemiology**

Median age at presentation is 60; mean survival after diagnosis (without treatment) is 30 months. More common in African Americans.

**Management**

Administer **systemic chemotherapy** (alkylating agents are used most commonly); bone lesions require **bisphosphonates** and **local radiation** to prevent pathologic fracture. Give **IV gamma-globulin** to correct profound hypogammaglobulinemia and reduce infections; **treat hypercalcemia;** manage pain; **bone marrow transplant** in refractory cases. Administer **pneumococcal vaccine.**

**Complications**

**Hyperviscosity syndrome** (visual and mental status disturbances, vertigo, headache, and mucosal bleeding), cryoglobulinemia, pathologic fractures (possibly leading to spinal cord compression, carpal tunnel syndrome, etc.), recurrent infections, sepsis, **amyloidosis, light-chain nephropathy** with renal failure, and peripheral neuropathy (due to amyloidosis).

**Breakout Point**

- Low back (bone) pain in elderly patient
- Plasma cell tumor: M spike from monoclonal paraprotein
- Punched-out lytic bone lesions
- Bence-Jones (light-chain) proteinuria
- Rouleaux formation and anemia
- Myeloma kidney

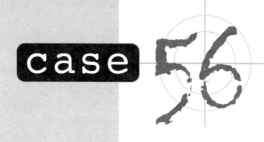

case 56

| | |
|---|---|
| **ID/CC** | A **61-year-old man** complains of **painless lumps** (LYMPHADENOPATHY) in his neck and groin that have been increasing in size. |
| **HPI** | He additionally reports **mild fever, weight loss,** and **night sweats** over the past 3 months. |
| **PE** | VS: low-grade fever (38.3°C). PE: pallor; cervical, axillary, and femoral lymphadenopathy; large mass in **Waldeyer ring; splenomegaly.** |
| **Labs** | CBC: Coombs-positive hemolytic **anemia;** thrombocytopenia. Elevated serum LDH; hypergammaglobulinemia. LP: no malignant cells in CSF. Lymph node dissection reveals lymphoid follicles throughout lymph node. |
| **Imaging** | CXR/CT, chest, pelvis, abdomen: lymphadenopathy and organ involvement; assess the spread of disease. |

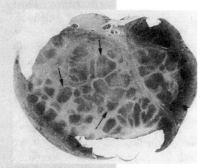

**Figure 56-1.** Lymph node dissection reveals lymphoid follicles throughout lymph node.

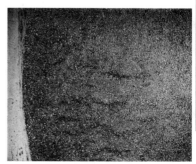

**Figure 56-2.** In another type of non-Hodgkin lymphoma, lymph nodes are diffusely infiltrated by lymphoma cells.

HEME/ONC

case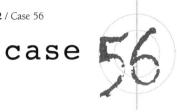

## Non-Hodgkin Lymphoma

**Pathogenesis**

Non-Hodgkin lymphomas are malignant neoplasms arising from lymphoid cells or other cells native to lymphoid tissue. They are classified on the basis of histopathologic cell type (small lymphocytic, follicular small cleaved, etc.). Staging of the disease is as follows. **Stage I:** involvement of a single lymph node region or extralymphatic site. **Stage II:** involvement of two or more lymph node areas on the same side of the diaphragm. **Stage III:** involvement of lymph node areas on both sides of the diaphragm (many include spleen). **Stage IV:** one or more extralymphatic organs (with or without lymphatic spread).

**Epidemiology**

**Small lymphocytic, follicular small-cell cleaved,** and **large-cell lymphomas** are most common in older adults. Individuals with HIV are particularly prone to immunoblastic lymphoma of the CNS. Lymphoblastic and small cell uncleaved lymphomas are most common in children.

**Management**

Staging (e.g., bone or gallium scan) and tumor histology direct treatment. Aggressive **combination chemotherapy** is the mainstay of treatment for high-grade lymphomas; **Rituximab** (a monoclonal antibody directed against the B-cell surface antigen CD20) has been administered in combination with chemotherapy. Surgery or radiation therapy may be required for large obstructive or bulky tumors. In general, patients with low-grade disease survive long but are rarely cured; high-grade tumors respond well to treatment and may be cured.

**Complications**

Complications include superior vena cava syndrome, metastasis, and bowel obstruction. Tumor lysis syndrome may cause hyperkalemia, hypocalcemia, hyperphosphatemia, and hyperuricemia. Common chemotherapeutic complications include bone marrow suppression, hemorrhagic cystitis (cyclophosphamide), cardiomyopathy (doxorubicin/Adriamycin), pulmonary fibrosis (bleomycin), peripheral neuropathy and weakness (vincristine), and hypertension (prednisone).

**Breakout Point**

- Includes a group of cancers: follicular small cell cleaved, Burkitt's small lymphocytic, large cell lymphomas

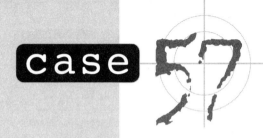

## case 57

**ID/CC** A **62-year-old white man** complains of increasing **headaches, dizziness,** and **fatigue** over the past month.

**HPI** The patient reports that his headaches have become more frequent and have been accompanied by **ringing in the ears** (TINNITUS) and **blurry vision.** The patient additionally notes **generalized itching** following warm showers (due to histamine release).

**PE** VS: hypertension. PE: **facial plethora; engorged retinal veins;** neurologic exam nonfocal; mild hepatomegaly; **splenomegaly.**

**Labs** CBC: **hematocrit elevated** (>60%); **elevated RBC mass; elevated WBC count** (13,000); mild basophilia; **thrombocytosis** (600,000). PBS: **normal RBC morphology.** ABGs: normal. **Low erythropoietin;** elevated vitamin $B_{12}$ levels (due to increased transcobalamin III levels); elevated leukocyte alkaline phosphatase; elevated uric acid.

**Imaging** None.

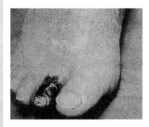

**Figure 57-1.** Gangrene attributable to vascular thrombosis (hyperviscosity).

# case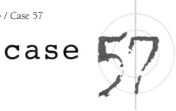

## Polycythemia Vera (PCV)

**Pathogenesis**

Polycythemia vera is an acquired **myeloproliferative disorder** that is characterized by overproduction of all three hematopoietic cell lines with predominant elevation in RBCs. This overproduction is **independent of erythropoietin**; a mutation in Jak2 may be the cause.

**Epidemiology**

Relatively common; seen more frequently in **males** (60%) and presents most commonly in late middle life (**median age 60** at presentation). The disease is uncommon among blacks.

**Management**

Periodic **phlebotomy** to reduce the hematocrit to <46%. Iron deficiency is inevitable in many patients with continued phlebotomy; iron supplementation may be required. **Myelosuppressive therapy** may be indicated if patients develop a high phlebotomy requirement, thrombocytosis, or intractable pruritus. **Hydroxyurea** achieves long-term disease control in most patients. Alkylating agents should be avoided because of leukemogenic potential. **Alpha-interferon** may be used in combination with intermittent phlebotomy or hydroxyurea in refractory patients. A reduction of platelet count to <600,000 reduces the risk of thrombotic complications; thus, patients may benefit from antiplatelet agents and/or anticoagulants. Antihistamines can be used to control pruritus.

**Complications**

Polycythemia vera has a median survival of 6 to 8 months untreated and 11 to 12 years with adequate therapy. Most complications, such as gangrene, are attributable to **vascular thrombosis** (hyperviscosity). Hemorrhage can result from **peptic ulcer formation** (dysfunctional platelets, increased histamine, and gastric acid production); **hyperuricemia** may result from increased cell turnover. Patients who reach the "spent" or "burnt-out" phase develop marked splenomegaly and anemia associated with bone marrow fibrosis.

**Breakout Point**

- Presents with symptoms related to hyperviscosity
- Primary polycythemia vera: low erythropoietin
- Secondary polycythemia vera: high erythropoietin

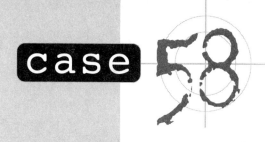

# case 58

| | |
|---|---|
| **ID/CC** | A **56-year-old man** presents to the clinic with **fatigue, weight loss,** and **night sweats.** |
| **HPI** | He has a 30-pack-year history of **smoking.** He also reports difficulty swallowing and hoarseness. |
| **PE** | VS: tachycardic. PE: engorged neck veins. |
| **Labs** | CBC: anemic (Hb 9). Lytes: decreased sodium. |
| **Imaging** | CT chest: large central pulmonary mass compressing esophagus. |

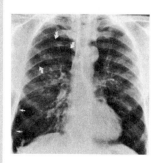

**Figure 58-1.** Superior vena cava occlusion by mass (*arrows*) in the right hilar region (bilateral upper extremity venogram).

# case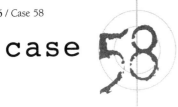

## Small-Cell Carcinoma of the Lung

**Pathogenesis**

Cumulative exposure to tobacco and other carcinogens causes genetic mutations that result in malignant transformation. **Small, round, blue neuroendocrine cells** compose these tumors. Nearly 90% of cases are linked to p53 mutations. Aggressive in nature, this form of cancer is usually only responsive to **chemotherapy and radiation,** (not surgery) since **disease is typically metastatic at time of diagnosis.** These tumors tend to occur centrally. Small-cell carcinoma is also associated with **paraneoplastic syndromes** of ACTH and ADH overexpression.

**Epidemiology**

Small-cell carcinoma accounts for 20% to 25% of all lung cancers and is the most aggressive of all lung tumors.

**Management**

Treatment **depends upon staging,** which is determined by tissue biopsy, CT, MRI, bone scans, and the TNM (tumor, node, metastasis) classification system. Treatment includes **chemotherapy** (cisplatin and etoposide) and **radiation.** **Surgical resection for small-cell carcinoma is ineffective** (unlike non-small-cell carcinoma). Patients presenting with limited stage (local nonbulky tumors) have a 15% to 20% cure rate with treatment.

**Complications**

Five-year survival rate is 15% for all lung cancers; small-cell carcinoma mean survival is only 1 year. Without treatment, there may only be a 6- to 17-week survival. These tumors have the highest propensity to **metastasize** and can cause debilitating syndromes.

**Breakout Point**

| Syndromes Associated with Small-Cell Lung Carcinoma |
| --- |
| 1. SIADH |
| 2. Lambert-Eaton syndrome (muscle weakness caused by autoantibodies) |
| 3. Horner syndrome (ptosis, miosis, anhydrosis caused by sympathetic ganglia damage) |
| 4. Superior vena cava syndrome (facial, neck, and arm swelling from tumor impingement on SVC) |
| 5. Cushing syndrome (ACTH) |

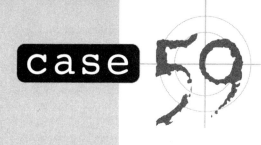

# case 59

**ID/CC** A **33-year-old Chinese woman** is found to have a low hematocrit on routine screening labs.

**HPI** The patient is otherwise healthy with no complaints. She recalls having had a previous bout with anemia during childhood but denies any hemoptysis, hematochezia, melena, menorrhagia, gross hematuria, or other bleeding tendencies. Her **brother had a similar anemia** in childhood and has always had "low blood."

**PE** VS: normal. PE: conjunctiva pale; no petechiae or ecchymoses noted; lung, cardiac, and abdominal exams normal; rectal exam normal with heme-negative stool.

**Labs** CBC/PBS: **low hemoglobin** (9.4 g/dL) **and hematocrit** (28.9%); microcytes; hypochromia; occasional target cells; **low MCV** (69). **Iron studies normal;** normal reticulocyte count; hemoglobin electrophoresis reveals **normal HgA and HgA$_2$.**

**Imaging** None.

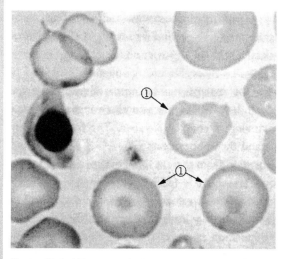

**Figure 59-1.** Microcytes; hypochromia; occasional target cells (*1*).

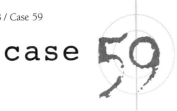

# case 59

## Thalassemia—Alpha

**Pathogenesis**

Thalassemia is a hereditary disorder that results from impaired production of globin chains (α or β) that leads to a defective hemoglobin structure within RBCs and to a hypochromic, microcytic anemia. **α-thalassemias** are due to **gene deletions** that directly cause reduced α-globin chain synthesis with no effect on HgA, HgA$_2$, or HgF structure. Excess β-chains in the severe form may produce a B4 tetramer (HgH). **β-thalassemias** are usually caused by **point mutations** that result in reduced or absent β-globin synthesis. Excess α-chains that are produced are unstable and can precipitate, thus damaging RBC membranes and causing intramedullary hemolysis and resultant bone marrow hyperplasia. Homozygous disease (thalassemia major) presents as severe transfusion-requiring anemia during the first year of life, usually manifesting after 6 months, when hemoglobin synthesis shifts from HgF to HgA.

**Epidemiology**

**α-thalassemias** are seen in individuals from Southeast Asia or China and, less commonly, in blacks. **β-thalassemia** usually affects individuals of Mediterranean origin (Greek or Italian).

**Management**

No treatment is indicated for asymptomatic α-thalassemia. **Regular transfusions** and **folate supplementation** are indicated for severe α-thalassemia (COOLEY ANEMIA). Patients with the HgH variant require transfusions only during acute hemolytic exacerbations. **Splenectomy** is performed when hypersplenism increases the requirement for more frequent transfusions. **Deferoxamine** is routinely offered as an iron-chelating agent to prevent or postpone hemosiderosis. **Allogeneic bone marrow transplantation** is now an option for α-thalassemic children who have not yet developed iron overload or chronic organ toxicity.

**Complications**

Untreated chronic iron overload secondary to thalassemia may result in **cardiomyopathy,** progressive hepatomegaly, and endocrine dysfunction. Death from **cardiac failure** may occur by the third decade.

**Breakout Point**

- Microcytosis out of proportion to clinical anemia
- Family history of microcytic anemia
- Hemoglobin H (beta4 tetramer) in severe disease

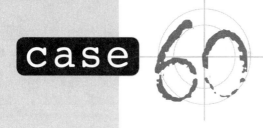

ID/CC A **28-year-old woman** is brought to the emergency room after having a **seizure** at work.

HPI The patient also complains of increased **fatigue.** She first noticed these symptoms several weeks ago but has only recently sought care.

PE VS: tachycardia (HR 126); hypertensive 170/80, **fever** (39.3°C). PE: pallor; multiple **petechiae;** no hepatosplenomegaly; neurologic examination normal.

Labs CBC/PBS: **thrombocytopenia** (53,000); **elevated reticulocyte count; schistocytes;** helmet cells; **altered platelet morphology.** LDH increased; PT/PTT normal; fibrinogen concentrations normal. Elevated BUN and creatinine. UA: proteinuria.

Imaging None.

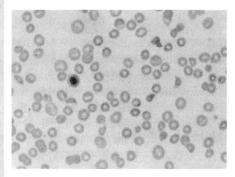

**Figure 60-1.** Peripheral blood smear demonstrating schistocytes.

HEME/ONC

# case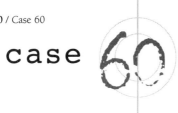

## Thrombotic Thrombocytopenic Purpura (TTP)

**Pathogenesis**

Thrombotic thrombocytopenic purpura (TTP) is characterized by the presence of **microangiopathic hemolytic anemia, thrombocytopenia, neurologic disorders, renal dysfunction,** and **fever.** Its precise etiology is unknown, but a strong immunologic component is suspected. Pathologically, localized arteriolar thrombi and fibrin deposition produce most disease manifestations.

**Management**

**Glucocorticoids,** splenectomy, and antiplatelet drugs are used with some success. Antiplatelet drugs (aspirin, dextran, dipyridamole, and sulfinpyrazone) may be used in conjunction with other treatments. Acute life-threatening complications require emergent exchange transfusion or **plasmapheresis** coupled with infusion of fresh frozen plasma. Patients are at risk of death or coma. Remission occurs in two-thirds of patients if treated promptly.

**Complications**

Patients may develop GI or GU hemorrhage, pancreatitis, progressive CNS dysfunction (delirium, confusion, seizure, aphasia, and visual field deficits), or renal failure. May be fatal. Relapses occur in 10% of cases.

**Breakout Point**

> Pentad: fever, anemia, thrombocytopenia, neurologic changes, and renal failure

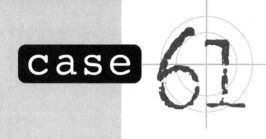

**case 61**

**ID/CC**
A **19-year-old woman** is referred by her dentist for evaluation of complaints of **easy bruising** and **bleeding.**

**HPI**
She has a history of **easy bruising** and frequent **nosebleeds** (epistaxis) since early childhood. She also reports a history of **heavy** (>10 pads per day) and **prolonged** (>7 days) **menses** since the onset of menarche. Her 12-year-old sister required blood transfusions after tonsillectomy several years ago. Her father bled for several days after a wisdom tooth extraction.

**PE**
VS: normal. PE: **conjunctivae** slightly **pale;** large (>4 cm) superficial **ecchymoses** on extremities.

**Labs**
CBC: mild microcytic anemia; **normal platelets.** Normal PT. **Prolonged aPTT. Prolonged bleeding time.** Decreased factor VIII activity. Reduced von Willebrand factor (vWF) level. **Decreased ristocetin cofactor activity.**

**Imaging**
None.

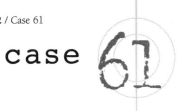

case

# von Willebrand Disease

**Pathogenesis**

Von Willebrand disease (vWD) is a heterogeneous group of bleeding disorders caused by **deficiency or dysfunction of vWF**. Most cases are **congenital** (autosomal dominant or recessive), but **acquired** forms of vWD may be caused by formation of autoantibodies against vWF or other mechanisms. The two major functions of vWF are (1) **to facilitate platelet adhesion and aggregation and** (2) **to act as a carrier for the circulating factor VIII**, preventing its degradation and prolonging its half-life. Because of vWF's role in platelet interactions, the clinical manifestations of vWD are generally similar to those seen in other platelet disorders (immediate mucocutaneous bleeding, easy bruising, menorrhagia, etc.). **Reduced factor VIII levels result in prolongation of aPTT** (see Table 61-1). Bleeding into joints and deep tissues (pseudohemophilia) is rare, but can occur in subtypes of vWD associated with very low factor VIII levels.

**Epidemiology**

vWD is the most common inherited bleeding disorder with estimated prevalence of up to 1% in the general population. Affects both sexes equally.

**Management**

Treat inherited vWD with **desmopressin** (except type 2b), **vWF-containing factor concentrates**, antifibrinolytic drugs, and topical thrombin. Estrogen may be used in some settings. Hormonal therapy for menorrhagia in women and iron supplementation are sometimes necessary. Avoid aspirin and other anti-platelet agents. For acquired vWD, the focus of therapy should be treatment of the underlying condition. IVIG is used in antibody-mediated acquired vWD.

**Complications**

<5% of cases are clinically significant.

**Breakout Point**

- Autosomal dominant inheritance
- Prolonged bleeding time
- Decreased factor VIII activity (vWF is a carrier protein for factor VIII)

■ TABLE 61-1 COMPARISON OF MAJOR FEATURES OF VON WILLEBRAND DISEASE AND HEMOPHILIA

|  | vWD | Hemophilia |
|---|---|---|
| Inheritance | Autosomal dominant (majority) or recessive | X-linked recessive (hemophilia A) |
| Symptoms | Mucocutaneous bleeding | Hemarthroses; deep tissue bleeding |
| Platelet count | Normal | Normal |
| Bleeding time (poor sensitivity and specificity) | May be prolonged | Normal |
| PT | Normal | Normal |
| aPTT | Prolonged/normal | Prolonged |
| Factor VIII activity | Decreased | Decreased |
| vWF antigen | Decreased | Normal |
| Ristocetin cofactor (vWF activity) | Decreased | Normal |

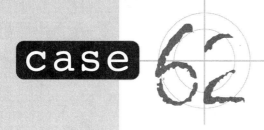

# case 62

| | |
|---|---|
| **ID/CC** | A **42-year-old obese woman** presents with one day of **right upper quadrant (RUQ) tenderness** and nausea. |
| **HPI** | Her pain has persisted over the past day and radiates to the **right shoulder.** She reports fevers, nausea, vomiting, and anorexia. She has had similar episodes in the past, especially after eating a fatty meal. |
| **PE** | VS: febrile. PE: abdomen is soft and obese with hypoactive bowel sounds; pain on palpation of RUQ and has inspiratory arrest with deep inspiration (**Murphy sign**). |
| **Labs** | CBC: leukocytosis (13,000) with a left shift. LFTs: mild ALT and AST elevation. |
| **Imaging** | **RUQ US: gallbladder wall thickening, pericholecystic fluid,** cholelithiasis with a **postacoustic shadow** (void behind the gallstones). She had pain when the ultrasound device was pressed on her gallbladder (**sonographic Murphy sign**). |

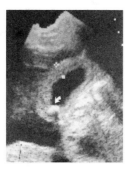

**Figure 62-1.** Marked thickening of the gallbladder neck (1.1 cm between the cursors). There is a densely echogenic stone (*arrow*) with posterior acoustic shadowing in the neck of the gallbladder.

# case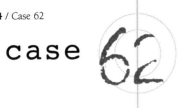

## Acute Cholecystitis

**Pathogenesis**

Acute cholecystitis is an **inflammation of the gall-bladder mucosa.** Approximately 90% of cases are associated with **cholelithiasis.** It is thought that a gallstone obstructing the cystic duct contributes to inflammation of the gallbladder mucosa. Acalculous cholecystitis (no stone is identified) occurs in 5% to 10% of patients with acute cholecystitis. Predisposing factors include parenteral nutrition, diabetes, vasculitis, trauma, and burns.

**Epidemiology**

The male-to-female ratio is 1:3 and the peak age of incidence is 40 to 60 years.

**Management**

Empiric therapy with antibiotics should be directed against **gram-negative bacteria (*Klebsiella, E. coli, Enterococcus,* and *Enterobacter*)** and anaerobes. There is a high risk of complications, so a cholecystectomy is usually performed after 24 to 48 hours of supportive therapy. Patients who are unstable or have complications may need emergent surgery.

**Complications**

Gangrene, perforation, empyema, and emphysematous cholecystitis.

**Breakout Point**

The 5 F's: A fertile, fat, flatulent female in her 40s.

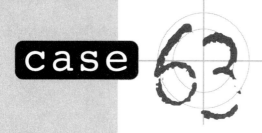

# case 63

**ID/CC**  A **35-year-old man** complains of severe **epigastric pain** radiating to his back for the past 2 hours.

**HPI**  He reports significant post-prandial abdominal pain, **nausea, and emesis** over past day. He feels more comfortable when leaning forward. Of note, the patient has a history of extensive alcohol intake with a noted binge 2 days ago.

**PE**  VS: hypertensive, tachycardic. PE: **sitting up and leaning forward;** abdomen exquisitely tender over the epigastric region with some rebound and guarding; **Cullen sign** (periumbilical ecchymosis) and **Grey–Turner sign** (flank ecchymosis) are negative (these signs indicate hemorrhagic pancreatitis).

**Labs**  CBC: macrocytic anemia. Lytes: metabolic acidosis. **Amylase and lipase increased.**

**Imaging**  CT abdomen: pancreatic calcifications with no pseudocyst or abscess. US right upper quadrant: no cholelithiasis.

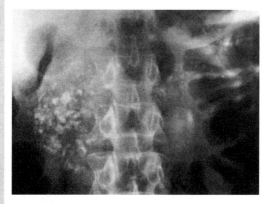

**Figure 63-1.** KUB: pancreatic calcifications.

case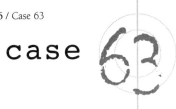

## Acute Pancreatitis

**Pathogenesis**

Pancreatitis most commonly originates due to a dysfunction in the synthesis and secretion of pancreatic digestive enzymes from exocrine cells. Usually synthesis continues while secretion is obstructed; this can be caused by a stone in the pancreatic duct or by inflammation of the duct. Digestive enzymes leak out of acinar cells and into the systemic circulation, causing serum amylase and lipase elevation. **Alcoholism and gallstones account for 70% of disease.** Certain drugs, such as **hydrochlorothiazide** or HIV medications such as **DDI,** can precipitate attacks. Trauma, recent ERCP, scorpion bites, hypertriglyceridemia, hypercalcemia, and viral illnesses such as mumps are less common etiologies.

**Epidemiology**

Age and gender are determined by etiology; alcoholism more common in males and cholelithiasis more common in females.

**Management**

**Ranson criteria and APACHE II score** determine severity and outcome. In less severe cases, supportive care with aggressive IVF resuscitation, bowel rest, and pain management is recommended. In patients with gallstones, cholecystectomy several weeks after the patient has stabilized is standard of care.

**Complications**

Pseudocyst, pancreatic insufficiency (diabetes and malabsorption), necrotizing pancreatitis, rarely retroperitoneal bleeding (Grey–Turner or Cullen sign is associated with a poor prognosis), shock, and death.

**Breakout Point**

- Pancreatitis is a clinical diagnosis
- Most common etiologies: alcoholism and gallstones
- Radiologic sign of chronic pancreatitis: pancreatic calcifications

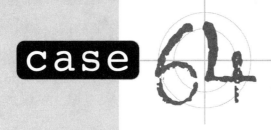

# case 64

| | |
|---|---|
| ID/CC | A **26-year-old woman** presents with **diarrhea** and weight loss for the past several months. |
| HPI | She reports that her stools have been **malodorous**. Other associated symptoms include **abdominal bloating, flatulence, cramps, fatigue, and generalized arthralgias**. |
| PE | VS: normal. PE: **very thin** woman in NAD with **pale conjunctiva** and an otherwise normal exam; stool negative for blood on rectal exam. |
| Labs | CBC: microcytic anemia. **Anti-TTG (tissue transglutaminase) IgA positive.** Iron: low. Ferritin: markedly decreased. Lytes: hypocalcemia. Pathology from duodenal biopsy: mucosal inflammation, crypt hyperplasia, and villous atrophy. |
| Imaging | EGD: scalloped duodenal folds. |

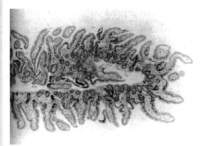

**Figure 64-1.** Normal gastrointestinal microvilli.

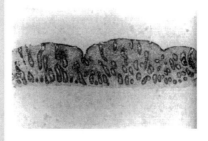

**Figure 64-2.** Flattened intestinal microvilli.

GI

# case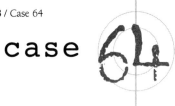

## Celiac Disease

**Pathogenesis**

Celiac disease is a **gluten-sensitive enteropathy** that results in a chronic inflammatory disorder. Gluten is commonly found in wheat, barley, and rye. HLA DR3 and DQw2 are two haplotypes commonly associated with this disorder. Inflammation due to gluten sensitivity leads to **atrophy of the small intestinal villi** and subsequent **malabsorption** with associated bulky, foul-smelling, floating stools due to steatorrhea, flatulence, weight loss, **iron-deficiency anemia,** neurologic disorders from deficiencies of B vitamins, and osteopenia from deficiency of vitamin D and calcium. There are several associated conditions including **dermatitis herpetiformis,** autoimmune thyroid disease, liver disease, and infertility.

**Epidemiology**

Celiac disease occurs primarily in whites of northern European ancestry.

**Management**

Treatment is **strict adherence to a gluten-free diet,** which is curative. The most common reasons for a lack of response are poor compliance or inadvertent gluten ingestion. For this reason, a good dietary history and involvement with a nutritionist early are important steps toward adequate treatment.

**Breakout Point**

- Gluten-free diet is curative
- May be diagnosed due to iron deficiency anemia
- Associated with dermatitis herpetiformis
- Villous atrophy and blunting

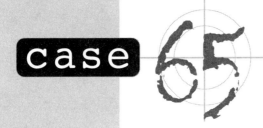

# case 65

**ID/CC** A **59-year-old man** with a history of **alcoholism** presents with **persistent upper abdominal** (EPIGASTRIC) **pain that radiates to the back.**

**HPI** The pain was **initially episodic** but is now **constant**, is not relieved by antacids, and is worsened by the ingestion of alcohol or fatty foods. The patient denies nausea or vomiting (versus acute pancreatitis), but states that he frequently has **foul-smelling, loose, bulky, greasy stool** (STEATORRHEA). He adds that he has lost 20 pounds over the past year.

**PE** VS: low-grade fever (38.2°C). PE: cachectic; jaundiced (secondary to edema and fibrosis at the head of the pancreas causing common bile duct obstruction); mild epigastric tenderness without rebound or rigidity.

**Labs** CBC/PBS: decreased hematocrit. Lytes: hypocalcemia, amylase and lipase normal; **decreased serum trypsinogen levels; reduced pancreatic enzyme secretion** on stimulation; stool exam reveals **increased fecal fat.**

**Imaging** See Figures 65-1 to 65-4.

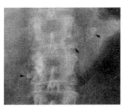

**Figure 65-1.** KUB. Multiple **calcifications** in the distribution of the pancreas.

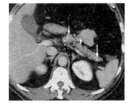

**Figure 65-2.** CT, abdomen. Punctate calcifications within the pancreas (*arrows*).

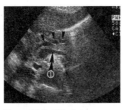

**Figure 65-3.** US, abdomen. "Chain of lakes" deformity of the pancreatic duct caused by many strictures with intervening areas of dilation (*arrows*); splenic vein (*1*).

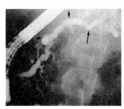

**Figure 65-4.** ERCP. A dilated and irregular pancreatic duct.

# case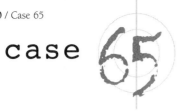

## Chronic Pancreatitis

**Pathogenesis**

Chronic pancreatitis is characterized by **extensive pancreatic fibrosis,** clinically presenting with pain, malabsorption, or repeated episodes of acute inflammation in a previously damaged pancreas. Causes include **alcoholism** (the most common cause of pancreatic exocrine insufficiency in adults in the United States), **cystic fibrosis** (the most common cause in children), or causes of **acute pancreatitis** (which lead to recurrent episodes of pancreatic inflammation, as seen in chronic relapsing pancreatitis); it may also be idiopathic.

**Epidemiology**

Alcohol-induced pancreatitis is more common in **males,** with an age of onset between 40 and 49 years. Some 5% to 10% of heavy alcohol users develop pancreatitis. Most cases in children are secondary to cystic fibrosis.

**Management**

Therapy is directed toward **eliminating the underlying cause, treating malabsorption, minimizing pain,** and **delaying disease progression.** Consequently, patients should be encouraged to maintain a low-fat diet and to **abstain from alcohol;** given **NSAIDs** or **narcotics** (long-term use should be avoided) for pain; and given vitamin supplements (fat-soluble vitamins and vitamin $B_{12}$) and **pancreatic enzymes** with antacids for malabsorption (enzymes are inactivated below a pH of 4). Patients who develop diabetes may require **insulin.** In cases of intractable pain, **surgery** should be considered.

**Complications**

Complications include diabetes mellitus, pancreatic exocrine insufficiency, pancreatic cancer, pancreatic pseudocyst or abscess (in acute exacerbations), common bile duct or duodenal obstruction, splenic vein thrombosis, ascites, and pleural effusion. Narcotic dependence may become an issue.

**Breakout Point**

- Epigastric pain, steatorrhea, weight loss
- Most common cause—alcoholism
- Prone to pseudocyst, abscess, or malignancy

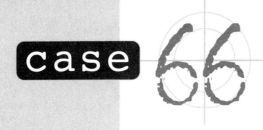
**ID/CC** A **78-year-old woman** presents with 10 pounds of **unintentional weight loss** and weakness for the past 3 months.

**HPI** She reports worsening pain and anorexia. Her husband noticed that she has become pale and increasingly fatigued. She denies changes in the caliber of her stool. Of note, the patient has a **history of iron deficiency anemia.**

**PE** VS: normal. PE: abdomen is soft with no rebound or guarding; guaiac positive brown stool; no palpable masses.

**Labs** CBC: microcytic anemia, hematocrit 21.

**Imaging** Colonoscopy reveals fungating mass which is biopsied.

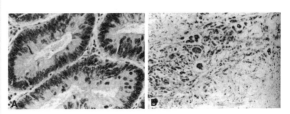

**Figure 66-1.** Histopathology of mass showing "back-to-back" glands.

# case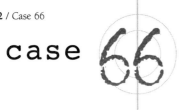

## Colon Cancer

**Pathogenesis**

Colon cancer is predominantly adenocarcinoma that arises from adenomatous polyps (**adenoma-carcinoma sequence**). Colon cancer is associated with mutations in tumor suppressor genes such as p53, Ki-RAS, or APC (adenomatous polyposis coli). APC is present in patients with **familial adenomatous polyposis,** who have a 100% chance of developing colon cancer.

**Epidemiology**

The risk of developing colon cancer is 7% and increases with age. Some risks include age, low-fiber diet, inflammatory bowel disorders, and genetic syndromes. Smoking is also a risk factor.

**Management**

Two classification systems are used for staging: the **TNM** (tumor, regional lymph node, and metastasis) and **Duke classifications. Treatment depends on staging.** Chemotherapy includes 5 fluorouracil (5-FU), leucovorin, and **bevacizumab** (Avastin) (humanized monoclonal antibody against vascular endothelial growth factor [VEGF]). **Surgery** involves hemicolectomy. Early diagnosis with fecal occult blood testing and screening colonscopy is an important strategy. Patients without any genetic predisposition should begin screening colonoscopy at age 50, and repeat every 10 years if normal.

**Complications**

**Bowel obstruction**, anemia, short gut syndrome, hepatic and bony metastasis, and death.

**Breakout Point**

- Right-sided colon cancer: microcytic anemia and heme-positive stools
- Left-sided colon cancer: obstruction, decreased stool caliber

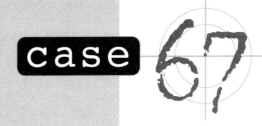

**ID/CC** A **24-year-old Jewish man** complains of persistent **nonbloody diarrhea.**

**HPI** The patient states that he has experienced fecal incontinence with small amounts of stool (perianal fistula). He has also had **colicky lower abdominal pain, weight loss, anorexia,** and periodic **joint pain.**

**PE** VS: fever (38.4°C); normal HR, RR, and BP. PE: thin and **pale** (secondary to anemia); temporal wasting; abdomen soft with **right lower quadrant tenderness and fullness;** no hepatosplenomegaly; orifice posterior to anus expresses stool (PERIANAL FISTULA).

**Labs** CBC: normal WBC; decreased hematocrit (28%). PBS: normochromic, normocytic RBCs. ESR elevated. LFTs: normal. Stool negative for ova and parasites; colonoscopy shows grossly inflamed colon with serpiginous ulcers separated by areas of normal mucosa (SKIP LESIONS); colonic biopsy reveals **noncaseating granuloma formation.**

**Imaging** See Figures 67-1 to 67-2.

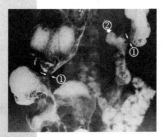

**Figure 67-1.** SBFT. A different case reveals two distinct areas of stricture formation (*1*) as well as a pseudodiverticulum (*2*).

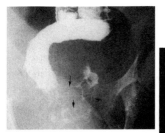

**Figure 67-2.** Barium enema: different case shows multiple fistulae between the rectum and vagina (*arrows*).

case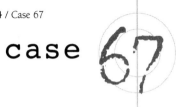

## Crohn Disease

**Pathogenesis**

The etiology of Crohn disease (regional enteritis) is unknown; however, several genetic, infectious, and immunologic theories have been advanced. It is characterized by **transmural inflammation that may affect any region extending from the mouth to the anus** (most commonly **terminal ileum**). Gross lesions appear as **serpiginous or linear ulcerations** with areas of intervening normal mucosa and **cobblestoning** with **stricture and fistula formation.** Histologically, they are classically seen as **noncaseating granulomas with crypt distortion and lymphocytic infiltration.**

**Epidemiology**

Crohn disease arises in approximately 0.1% of the population and in approximately 17% of individuals with an affected first-degree relative. The disease presents most commonly in the **third decade,** but a second peak in incidence arises in those aged 50 to 65. It occurs with the highest frequency in **Jewish men** (relative risk six times that of normal).

**Management**

Suppress disease activity with **corticosteroids** and **sulfasalazine** (or other 5-ASA derivatives). Antibiotic therapy (ciprofloxacin or metronidazole) can be given to patients who do not respond to aminosalicylates. **Immunosuppressive agents** (methotrexate, mercaptopurine, and/or azathioprine) may be used for refractory disease. Consider infliximab (anti-TNF antibody) in resistant cases. Patients may require vitamin $B_{12}$ injections and increased levels of calcium and vitamin D. Surgery, including **stricturoplasty** and/or **resection,** is indicated in cases of recurrent obstruction, enterocutaneous fistulas, intra-abdominal abscess, and disease refractory to medical therapy.

**Complications**

Intestinal obstruction, perforated viscus, intra-abdominal abscess, erythema nodosum, pyoderma gangrenosum, episcleritis, uveitis, peripheral arthritis, fistulas, malabsorption, and renal oxalate stones. Crohn disease is not associated with as significant an increase in cancer risk as ulcerative colitis, although patients are at increased risk when compared with normal patients.

**Breakout Point**

- Presents with colicky abdominal pain, fever, nonbloody diarrhea
- Anal skin tags and perianal fistulas
- Cobblestoning on colonoscopy

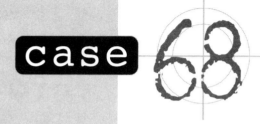

# case 68

**ID/CC** A **71-year-old woman** presents to the emergency room with painless **bright red blood per rectum** (HEMATOCHEZIA).

**HPI** She states that she frequently feels **constipated** and strains on defecation. She reports that her diet is **low in fiber.**

**PE** VS: no fever; tachycardia (HR 120); tachypnea (RR 20); normal BP. PE: alert and oriented; **pallor;** cool extremities; prolonged capillary refill; abdomen soft, nontender, and nondistended; positive bowel sounds; **bright red blood in rectal vault.**

**Labs** CBC: normal WBC; depressed hemoglobin (8.0 g/dL) and hematocrit (24%); normal platelets. Coagulation studies normal; nasogastric tube negative for blood or bile.

**Imaging** BE: **outpouchings of the sigmoid colon.**

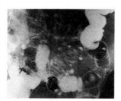

**Figure 68-1.** Barium enema. Multiple diverticula are seen as outpouchings of the sigmoid colon.

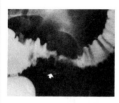

**Figure 68-2.** BE. A different case demonstrates a colonic stricture surrounded on both sides by many outpouchings of the colon.

# case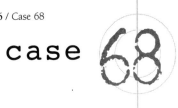

## Diverticulosis

**Pathogenesis**

Diverticula occur as a result of **high intraluminal pressure** distributed throughout a narrow lumen (such as the sigmoid colon), causing **herniations that lack a muscularis** (FALSE DIVERTICULA). The sigmoid is the most commonly affected segment. Diverticula typically **arise at sites where arterioles traverse the colonic wall** and are thus prone to bleeding. These outpouchings may also become obstructed, permitting growth of bacteria and consequent inflammation (DIVERTICULITIS).

**Epidemiology**

Colonic diverticula occur in approximately 33% of individuals older than 40 years and in **>50% of individuals older than 70 years.** Risk factors include a **low-fiber diet** (and therefore low stool weight) and living in a developed country.

**Management**

**High-fiber diet** and **transfusion for significant blood loss.** In cases of severe hemorrhage, mesenteric angiography is diagnostic and therapeutic (with intra-arterial embolization). In cases of recurrent diverticular bleeding or diverticulitis, patients should consider sigmoidectomy with a primary colorectal anastomosis. Diverticulitis is managed with broad-spectrum antibiotics with anaerobic coverage.

**Complications**

**Exsanguinating hemorrhage** is associated with untreated diverticular bleeds. Diverticulitis may lead to **abscess formation, peritonitis, fistula formation, and perforation.**

**Breakout Point**

- Presents as painless bright red blood per rectum
- Outpouchings of the colon

# case 69

**ID/CC** A **50-year-old woman** complains of **heartburn** and **burping** exacerbated by eating.

**HPI** She states that her symptoms occur approximately 30 to 60 minutes after meals and are **worsened when she lies down.** She has a 40-pack-year **smoking** history and is currently being treated with **diltiazem** for hypertension.

**PE** VS: mild hypertension (BP 146/88). PE: epigastrium tender on deep palpation.

**Labs** None.

**Imaging** Barium swallow: hiatal hernia and refluxed barium into hiatus. Endoscopically obtained mucosal biopsies (from 5 cm above the lower esophageal sphincter): changes of chronic esophagitis.

# case 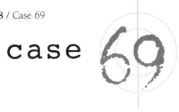 69

## Gastroesophageal Reflux Disease

**Pathogenesis**

Gastroesophageal reflux disease (GERD) is most often the result of toxic damage to the esophageal lining secondary to gastric acid exposure due to an incompetent lower esophageal sphincter.

**Epidemiology**

Risk factors for reflux include hiatal hernia, incompetent lower esophageal sphincter (LES), obesity, pregnancy, and scleroderma.

**Management**

Treatment focuses on **decreasing acid production (proton pump inhibitors, H₂ receptor antagonists), improving LES tone,** and increasing gastric motility **(metoclopramide).** Intervention should include **smoking cessation,** education on proper use of antacids, elevation of the head of the bed during sleep, **dietary restriction** (alcohol, mints, chocolate, fat, and caffeine), avoidance of meals 2 to 3 hours before sleep, and weight loss. Medications that decrease LES tone (e.g., calcium-channel blockers) should be avoided. Consider **surgery** (fundoplication, repair of hiatal hernia) for those who have not responded to medical therapy and lifestyle modification. Regular endoscopic surveillance should be conducted to rule out Barrett esophagus and adenocarcinoma.

**Complications**

Esophageal stricture, chronic aspiration, asthma, bleeding, and **Barrett esophagus** (a risk factor for adenocarcinoma).

**Breakout Point**

- Presents as burning epigastric pain or cough
- Can lead to Barrett esophagus, which can lead to adenocarcinoma

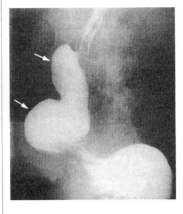

**Figure 69-1.** Barium swollen. Hiatal hernia and refluxed barium into hiatus.

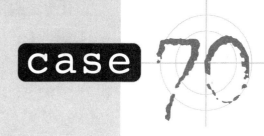

**ID/CC** A **50-year-old white man** presents with progressive **jaundice**, a peculiar skin rash, and joint pains; he also complains of generalized **fatigue** and muscle weakness.

**HPI** The jaundice has progressively worsened over the past 2 years. On directed questioning, the patient notes a decrease in libido and complains of pain in the knee and MCP joints of both hands. He has been diagnosed with **hyperglycemia** (BRONZE DIABETES) and dilated cardiomyopathy with atrial fibrillation. He does not smoke or drink alcohol.

**PE** VS: irregularly irregular pulse. PE: **bronze discoloration** seen diffusely, especially in sun-exposed areas; icterus; loss of pubic and axillary hair; testicular atrophy; spider nevi noted on chest and upper back; **liver enlarged** 5 cm below right costal margin; liver firm, nontender, and nonpulsatile; left knee swollen and tender.

**Labs** Elevated blood glucose; decreased serum testosterone and **gonadotropins;** increased serum iron; decreased TIBC; transferrin saturation >80%; **serum ferritin elevated** (>1,000 μg/L; best screening method). LFTs: elevated bilirubin; elevated AST and ALT; mildly elevated alkaline phosphatase. **Liver biopsy** shows high levels of stainable iron. ECG: atrial fibrillation (iron deposition in the heart with disruption of conduction pathways). Genetic testing for HFE mutation positive.

**Imaging** XR, knee: characteristic meniscal cartilage calcification (chondrocalcinosis). US, abdomen: liver with diffuse parenchymal infiltration suggestive of hepatitis. Echo: dilated cardiomyopathy.

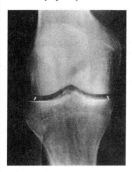

**Figure 70-1.** XR, knee. Characteristic meniscal cartilage calcification.

case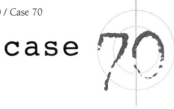

## Hemochromatosis

**Pathogenesis**

Hemochromatosis is an autosomal recessive disease characterized by excessive deposition of iron in parenchymal cells; it is due to a missense mutation in the **HFE gene** located on chromosome 6 and is caused by an **inappropriate increase** in **iron absorption** from the GI tract (normally, the amount of iron accumulated inversely affects GI mucosal absorption of both heme and nonheme iron). As iron overload progresses, iron that is ordinarily stored in the cells of the reticuloendothelial system is **deposited in the liver, joints, pituitary, pancreas, heart**, and **skin**. This pattern of deposition reflects the density of transferrin receptors in these tissues.

**Epidemiology**

Hemochromatosis is the most common single gene disorder of people of Caucasian descent. Most patients have HLA-A3 antigens. Despite an equal frequency of homozygosity, **males express clinical symptoms 10 times more often than females**; this may be due to regular menstrual and childbirth-associated blood loss in women.

**Management**

**Regular phlebotomy**; symptomatic management of joint and cardiac disease. **Deferoxamine** can be used in primary and in secondary iron overload. Continue treatment until serum studies normalize or anemia develops. Dietary modifications include avoidance of red meat, raw shellfish, alcohol, vitamin C, and supplemental iron. **Screen all first-degree relatives** with genetic testing for the HFE mutation. Cirrhosis may require transplantation.

**Complications**

**Heart failure, cirrhosis, hypogonadism, pancreatic insufficiency**, and **hepatocellular carcinoma** occur in end-stage disease.

**Breakout Point**

- Bronzing of the skin
- Diabetes from toxic iron deposits in the pancreas
- Bronze diabetes
- Liver insufficiency
- MCP joint arthropathy

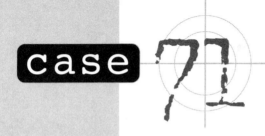

# case 71

**ID/CC**  A **47-year-old man** complains of **lack of appetite** (ANOREXIA), **weakness**, malaise, and **increasing abdominal girth** (ASCITES).

**HPI**  He also complains of marked **weight loss, impotence,** tea-colored urine, and passage of black, tarry, foul-smelling stools (MELENA). He was hospitalized a few weeks ago for treatment of **hematemesis**. He is a **heavy drinker**.

**PE**  VS: tachycardia (HR 105). PE: **muscle wasting**; mild **jaundice**; pallor; loss of axillary, chest, and pubic hair; enlargement of parotid glands; **palmar erythema; gynecomastia; spider nevi** in abdominal skin; caput medusae; **liver markedly enlarged** with a hard and nodular consistency (liver is small in end-stage cirrhosis); **splenomegaly**; positive fluid wave sign (due to ascites); testicular atrophy; pedal edema.

**Labs**  CBC: **macrocytic anemia; thrombocytopenia.** Prolonged PT. LFTs: AST/ALT ratio >2:1 (typical of alcoholic hepatic damage); elevated alkaline phosphatase; elevated GGT; elevated **bilirubin.** High blood ammonia; low BUN; low serum albumin; liver biopsy (CT-guided) reveals destruction of normal architecture with **regenerating nodules** and **fibrotic** changes; UGI endoscopy reveals presence of esophageal varices.

**Imaging**  UGI: filling defects in **"string of beads"** pattern (esophageal varices). CT, abdomen: the liver is seen to be shrunken and irregular, with a regenerative nodule in the caudate lobe; splenomegaly with multiple perisplenic varices is also seen.

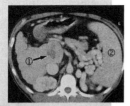

**Figure 71-1.** CT, abdomen. The liver is seen to be shrunken and irregular, with a regenerative nodule in the caudate lobe (*1*); splenomegaly with multiple perisplenic varices (*2*) is also seen.

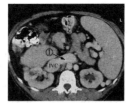

**Figure 71-2.** CT, abdomen. A different case shows not only splenomegaly but also dilatation of the left renal vein (*1*) and inferior vena cava (both the result of portosystemic shunting.

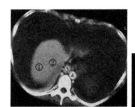

**Figure 71-3.** CT, abdomen. A different case demonstrates massive ascites (*3*); note the shrunken liver (*1*) and dilated inferior vena cava (*2*).

# case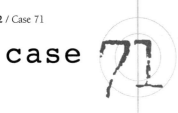

## Hepatic Cirrhosis

**Pathogenesis**

Cirrhosis is pathologically characterized by diffuse, irreversible, widespread hepatic parenchymal fibrosis in association with the formation of regenerative nodules. It is caused by **alcohol**, viruses (hepatitis B and C), primary biliary cirrhosis, extrahepatic biliary obstruction, hemochromatosis, $\alpha_1$-antitrypsin deficiency, cystic fibrosis, schistosomiasis, and Wilson disease. Histologically, it is divided into two variants: **macronodular** (POSTNECROTIC; usually associated with viral hepatitis) and **micronodular** (LAËNNEC; typically associated with alcohol).

**Epidemiology**

Cirrhosis is the ninth leading cause of death in the United States. It also predisposes patients to hepatocellular carcinoma. Thirty percent of patients with cirrhosis die within 1 year of diagnosis.

**Management**

**Cessation of alcohol use** is key. Hemorrhagic complications are managed with vitamin K and fresh frozen plasma. Ascites is managed with large-volume paracentesis, **salt and protein restriction,** and **diuretics** (spironolactone in combination with furosemide). Encephalopathy due to liver failure responds to decreased protein intake and **neomycin** and **lactulose** (to decrease serum ammonia). Spontaneous bacterial peritonitis is treated with IV antibiotics. Variceal bleeding may require **sclerotherapy,** transjugular intrahepatic portosystemic shunt (TIPS), or **surgical anastomosis.** Liver transplantation may be indicated.

**Complications**

Encephalopathy, variceal bleeding, portal vein thrombosis, hypersplenism, liver failure, hepatorenal syndrome, nutritional deficiencies, coagulopathy, and spontaneous bacterial peritonitis.

**Breakout Point**

- Regenerating nodules and fibrosis in liver
- Portal hypertension
- In case of hypotension or GI bleeding, suspect esophageal varices

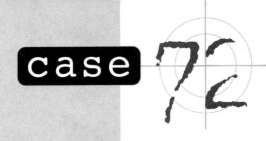

# case 72

**ID/CC** A **19-year-old man** complains of headache, **malaise,** nausea, vomiting, **loss of appetite,** and **fever** with chills for the past week.

**HPI** He also complains of passing **dark-colored urine** and clay-colored stool. He recently returned from a trip to a developing country where he ate shellfish from a street vendor.

**PE** VS: fever (39.2°C); mild tachycardia (HR 105); normal BP. PE: **icterus; tender hepatomegaly.**

**Labs** CBC: normal. LFTs: **AST and ALT markedly increased;** mild elevation in alkaline phosphatase and bilirubin. **Anti-HAV IgM present.**

**Imaging** None.

# case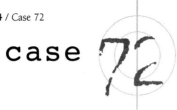

## Hepatitis A

**Pathogenesis**

The causative agent is hepatitis A virus (HAV), an RNA virus of the picornavirus family; it is transmitted by the **fecal–oral route** and produces an acute viral hepatitis. Unlike hepatitis B and C virus infections, **chronic hepatitis A infection does not occur.** Anti-HAV IgG confers immunity.

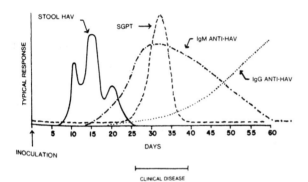

**Figure 72-1.** Course of hepatitis A infection.

**Epidemiology**

HAV transmission is enhanced by poor personal hygiene, contaminated food, and certain sexual practices. **No HAV carrier state has been identified,** and inapparent subclinical infection maintains the virus in nature. Affected children are often asymptomatic, with more severe disease typically occurring in adults.

**Management**

**No specific treatment. Rest** during the acute phase. Hospitalization may be required for severely ill patients. Alcohol, high fat intake, and drugs that produce adverse effects on the liver or require liver metabolism should be avoided. Give **hepatitis A and B vaccine** to travelers to endemic areas, patients with chronic liver disease, homosexual men, and animal handlers. **Hepatitis A immune globulin** is available for postexposure prophylaxis of all close personal contacts.

**Complications**

Relapse occurs only rarely but remains self-limited. Rare complications include myocarditis, cholestatic hepatitis, pancreatitis, aplastic anemia, atypical pneumonia, transverse myelitis, and peripheral neuropathy. Fulminant hepatitis is very rare; risk factors include increasing age and chronic liver disease.

**Breakout Point**

- Risk factors are foreign travel, occupation (daycare), and contaminated shellfish or water
- HAV IgM antibody indicates acute infection
- HAV IgG antibody indicates past infection and/or vaccination

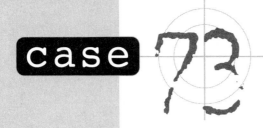

# case 73

**ID/CC**  A **49-year-old man** presents with **anorexia,** nausea, vomiting, and **jaundice.**

**HPI**  He also reports **pain** in his right upper quadrant and darkening of his urine. He has been a **heavy drinker** for the past 5 years and recently went on a week-long alcohol binge.

**PE**  VS: normal. PE: jaundice; tender hepatomegaly.

**Labs**  CBC: macrocytic anemia (due to folate deficiency); thrombocytopenia. Prolonged PT. LFTs: **AST and ALT elevated with >2:1 ratio;** elevated bilirubin, GGT, and alkaline phosphatase. Liver biopsy (CT-guided) reveals hepatocyte necrosis, Mallory bodies, infiltration of neutrophils, and perivenular fibrosis; UGI (endoscopy) reveals no esophageal varices but shows superficial gastric erosions with small petechiae.

**Imaging**  None.

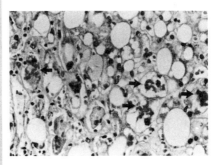

**Figure 73-1.** Mallory bodies (*arrows*) are evident within the swollen, clear cytoplasm of several hepatocytes.

GI

case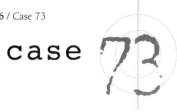

## Hepatitis, Alcoholic

**Pathogenesis**

The **amount and duration of alcohol consumption** are directly related to the development of alcoholic hepatitis. Initially, consumption of alcohol leads to the deposition of fat within hepatocytes. This leads to neutrophilic infiltration, hepatocyte **necrosis**, and collagen deposition in perivenular spaces and eventually to **cirrhosis.**

**Epidemiology**

Alcoholic liver disease affects >2 million Americans (i.e. approximately 1% of the population). Alcohol abuse is the most common cause of serious liver disease in Western societies. Risk factors for alcoholism include male gender, family history, regular drinking prior to age 16, Native American heritage, psychiatric illness, and antisocial personality.

**Management**

Therapy is initially directed toward **cessation of alcohol** and **management of complications** of the illness, such as variceal bleeding. Corticosteroids may decrease short-term mortality. Treat alcohol withdrawal; give nutritional support and vitamin supplements (including $B_{12}$, thiamine, and folate).

**Complications**

Complications include cirrhosis, which in turn predisposes patients to hepatocellular carcinoma, variceal bleeding, encephalopathy, and ultimately death. Nutritional deficiencies may produce Wernicke's encephalopathy (confusion, ataxia, ophthalmoplegia) resulting from thiamine deficiency. Long-term thiamine deficiency results in Wernicke–Korsakoff syndrome (a chronic amnestic disorder characterized by confabulation).

**Breakout Point**

- Quadrad of fever, RUQ pain, tender hepatomegaly, and jaundice
- AST:ALT is > 2:1
- Mallory bodies are characteristic histology finding

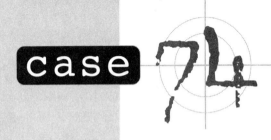

case 74

| | |
|---:|:---|
| **ID/CC** | A **49-year-old man** complains of yellow skin, yellow eyes, and mild right upper quadrant abdominal pain for 2 weeks. |
| **HPI** | The patient is a chronic alcoholic who used IV drugs for a year, until 2 weeks ago, when he became anorexic and nauseated. |
| **PE** | VSS. PE: **jaundice; scleral icterus;** mild (4/10) **RUQ abdominal pain.** |
| **Labs** | CBC: Mild thrombocytopenia; ALT 600 and AST 1250; total bilirubin 5.2; direct bilirubin 0.4; PT 30; PTT 45; INR 1.4. HepBSAg positive. Anti-HBc IgM positive, IgG negative. HBeAg positive. |
| **Imaging** | RUQ US: mild cirrhosis, no ascites; no gallstones or duct dilatation. |

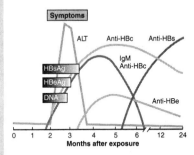

**Figure 74-1.** Course of hepatitis B infection.

# case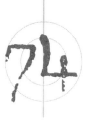

## Hepatitis B

**Pathogenesis**

Hepatitis B virus is a double-stranded DNA virus. HBV can cause direct cytotoxic liver injury; however, in most cases, HBV-related liver disease is related to cytotoxic T-cell–mediated lysis of infected hepatocytes. Both T-cell and antibody responses to HBV help control the infection. In general, there is no direct correlation between viral load or LFT elevation and the severity of disease. **Hepatitis B surface antigen (HBsAg) is the serologic hallmark of an HBV infection.** HBsAg appears in serum 1 to 10 weeks after an acute exposure to HBV, prior to the onset of hepatitic symptoms. In patients who subsequently recover, HBsAg usually becomes undetectable after 4 to 6 months. **Persistence of HBsAg for more than 6 months implies chronic infection.** Hepatitis B core antigen (HBcAg) is an intracellular antigen that is expressed in infected hepatocytes. It is not detectable in serum. **Anti-HBc antibody** can be detected throughout the course of HBV infection. Hepatitis Be antigen **(HBeAg) is a marker of HBV replication and infectivity.** The presence of HBeAg is usually associated with high levels of HBV DNA in serum. **Anti-HBs antibody confers protective immunity and is detected in patients who have recovered from HBV infection or who have received the HBV vaccine.**

**Epidemiology**

**Hepatitis B virus infection is a global public health problem. It is estimated that there are more than 300 million HBV carriers in the world, of whom approximately 500,000 die annually from HBV-related liver disease.** Perinatal transmission is most common in high prevalence areas such as Southeast Asia, while high-risk sexual behavior and IV drug use are most common in the United States, Canada, and Western Europe.

**Management**

Treatment strategies for chronic HBV include **interferon and antivirals.**

**Complications**

The sequelae of chronic HBV infection vary from an inactive carrier state to the development of **cirrhosis, hepatocellular carcinoma,** extrahepatic manifestations, and death.

**Breakout Point**

- HBsAg = marker of infection
- HBcAb = marker of window period or immunity
- HBeAg = a marker of HBV replication and infectivity
- HBsAb = marker of immunity or vaccination

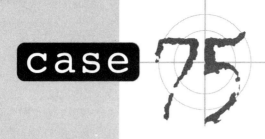

case 75

ID/CC A 22-year-old woman complains of colicky abdominal pain and diarrhea that occur 10 minutes after she starts eating.

HPI She also complains of a bloated sensation with lower abdominal distention that is more marked in the late afternoon. She reports increasing stress secondary to job pressure. She denies having any fever, weight loss, or nocturnal diarrhea.

PE VS: normal. PE: appears well nourished; no pallor, cyanosis, or jaundice; abdomen mildly distended, tympanic, and tender in hypogastrium; no masses or peritoneal signs; hyperactive bowel sounds.

Labs CBC/Lytes: normal. LFTs: normal. UA: normal. No occult blood in feces; stool ova and parasites negative; TFTs normal; sigmoidoscopy normal.

Imaging None.

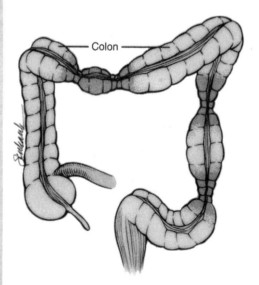

**Figure 75-1.** Altered GI motility.

GI

case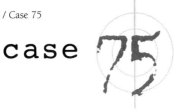

## Irritable Bowel Syndrome

**Pathogenesis**

Also called **spastic colitis** or nervous colitis, it is an idiopathic, **functional** intestinal motility disorder with a strong **relationship to stress**, anxiety, and depression.

**Epidemiology**

Irritable bowel syndrome is one of the most common GI disorders. The disorder shows a **female predominance**, generally starts prior to age 35 years, and is typically associated with a wide array of other "**psychosomatic**" **diseases**. The Rome III criteria for diagnoses require patients must have recurrent abdominal pain or discomfort at least 3 days per month during the previous 3 months that is associated with two or more of the following: relieved by defecation; onset associated with change in stool frequency; onset associated with change in stool form or appearance.

**Management**

**Reassurance**; psychiatric counseling; **high-fiber diet** low in irritants and gas-producing foods. Diphenoxylate and atropine/loperamide (for diarrhea) or psyllium/mild laxatives (for constipation); antidepressants, anxiolytics, or prokinetic drugs.

**Complications**

An increased incidence of **diverticulosis** is caused by prolonged constipation. Major psychological comorbidity also results in "doctor shopping" and dependency on narcotics or benzodiazepines.

**Breakout Point**

- Presents as abdominal discomfort with diarrhea or constipation
- Diagnosis of exclusion

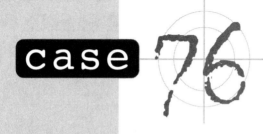

case 76

**ID/CC**  A **70-year-old man** presents with increasing **epigastric pain** for the past week.

**HPI**  He reports significant epigastric and left-sided abdominal pain that started suddenly 1 week ago and that **occurs 15 to 60 minutes after eating.** He has had a few episodes of **bright red blood per rectum** over the past day. He has a history of **atrial fibrillation** and has not been taking anticoagulants.

**PE**  VS: hypotension (BP 80/50) and tachycardia. PE: **patient in significant discomfort,** but abdomen is only mildly diffusely tender without rebound or guarding; maroon guaiac positive stool in the vault.

**Labs**  CBC: normocytic anemia.

**Imaging**  CT abdomen: **pneumatosis intestinalis** (air within the bowel wall), thromboembolism in the mesenteric vessels with irregular narrowing of the bowel lumen. Colonoscopy reveals pale colonic mucosa with extensive sloughing and ulceration. Barium enema demonstrates spasm with thickening and blunting of mucosal folds.

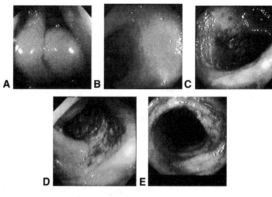

**Figure 76-1.** Colonoscopy. Pale colonic mucosa with extensive sloughing and ulceration.

GI

# case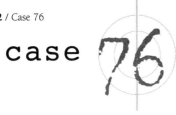

## Ischemic Colitis/Mesenteric Ischemia

**Pathogenesis**

Ischemic colitis is defined as insufficient blood supply to a bowel segment. Etiologies include **atherosclerosis, embolism, thrombosis, vasculitis, hypercoagulable states, and hypoperfusion during shock or congestive heart failure.** Occlusion of the superior mesenteric artery (SMA) may only affect the small bowel which is entirely dependent on mesenteric blood supply, while the large bowel can acquire a collateral posterior blood supply. Two **watershed territories of the colon** that are particularly vulnerable to ischemia include the **splenic flexure** between the SMA and inferior mesenteric artery (IMA) supply, and the **distal sigmoid colon** between the IMA and hypogastric artery supply. **Pneumatosis intestinalis** related with ischemia may be due to mucosal disruption, which allows bacteria or gas to enter the bowel wall, leading to bowel necrosis.

**Epidemiology**

Typically occurs in elderly patients with vascular disease, atherosclerosis, or atrial fibrillation (embolism risk).

**Management**

**CT abdomen** is the radiographic test of choice for diagnosis. **Angiography** showing abrupt cutoff of the SMA with no collaterals is the **gold standard for diagnosis,** but may not be appropriate for acutely ill patients who may require emergency surgical care. Treatment is determined by clinical status. For nonocclusive ischemia, **papaverine** (opium alkaloid which decreases visceral spasm) and supportive care with fluid resuscitation, antibiotics, bowel rest, and a lipid-lowering agent suffices. For acute arterial or venous embolism or thrombosis, **embolectomy, thrombolytics, or surgical bypass grafting** are recommended. Chronic mesenteric ischemia may benefit from **angioplasty or stenting** of the mesenteric vessels.

**Complications**

Can be life-threatening due to bowel necrosis, strictures, and sepsis.

**Breakout Point**

- Occlusion of mesenteric vessels leading to bowel necrosis in elderly patients
- Pain out of proportion to physical exam is the hallmark

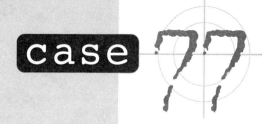

# case 77

| | |
|---|---|
| **ID/CC** | A **42-year-old man** business executive complains of **recurrent dyspepsia** over the past month. |
| **HPI** | The patient reports **epigastric discomfort** that he describes as gnawing, dull, achy, intermittent, episodic, that is **relieved by food or antacids.** He acknowledges a high-stress lifestyle with frequent business travel; he also **smokes** two packs of cigarettes per day and drinks heavily. |
| **PE** | VS: normal. PE: abdomen soft; mild tenderness to deep palpation in midepigastrium; no occult blood in stool. |
| **Labs** | CBC: hematocrit normal. Rapid urease breath test positive; serum *Helicobacter pylori* antibody positive; gastric mucosal biopsy reveals *H. pylori* infection; no evidence of malignancy. |
| **Imaging** | See Figures 77-1 to 77-4. |

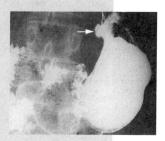

**Figure 77-1.** UGI. A barium-filled ulcer crater (*arrow*) is seen on the lesser curvature of the stomach.

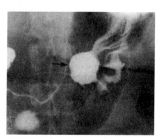

**Figure 77-2.** UGI. A large ulcer crater (*arrow)* is seen in the body of the stomach.

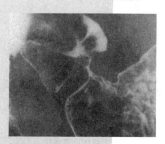

**Figure 77-3.** UGI. A different case showing multiple ulcers in the duodenum.

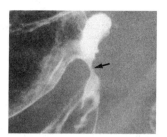

**Figure 77-4.** UGI. Scarring and stricture (*arrow*) formation in the duodenum secondary to long-standing peptic ulcer disease is seen in another case; note the stomach.

153

GI

# case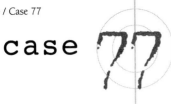

## Peptic Ulcer Disease

**Pathogenesis**

Peptic ulcers represent breaks in the gastric or duodenal mucosa that arise when normal mucosal defenses are compromised or are overwhelmed by acid and pepsin. *Helicobacter pylori* (a small, microaerophilic, **urease-producing**, gram-negative bacillus) has a close etiologic association with virtually all (95% to 100%) duodenal ulcer cases and most (75% to 85%) gastric ulcer cases. Other contributing factors include **NSAIDs, smoking, alcohol, aspirin, steroids, and stress**; duodenal ulcers are virtually always associated with a hyperacidic state. **Gastric ulcers should be biopsied** because up to 3% to 5% of even benign-appearing lesions prove to be malignant. Nonhealing ulcers are particularly suspicious for malignancy. Gastric malignancy is typically located in the bulb, pyloric channel, or greater curvature, whereas gastric ulcers are most commonly found in the antrum (60%) or the lesser curvature at the antrum-body junction (20%).

**Epidemiology**

Peptic ulcer disease has a lifetime prevalence of approximately 10% in the U.S. adult population. Duodenal ulcers are five times more common than gastric ulcers. Ulcers are slightly more common in men than in women. Duodenal ulcers tend to occur from 35 to 55 years of age, whereas gastric ulcers tend to occur from 55 to 70 years of age.

**Management**

Therapy is directed toward **ulcer healing and eradication of H. pylori.** *H. pylori*-associated ulcer disease is treated with a 10- to 14-day **triple therapy (amoxicillin, clarithromycin, proton-pump inhibitor). NSAIDs should be avoided.** Antacids and $H_2$-blockers are useful adjuncts. All patients with gastric ulcers or those whose symptoms persist despite adequate therapy should undergo endoscopy with biopsy after 6 to 12 weeks to rule out malignancy. Patients with severe recurring ulcers should have a serum gastrin level checked to rule out Zollinger–Ellison syndrome (gastrinoma).

**Complications**

Hemorrhage, perforation, gastric outlet obstruction, and gastric carcinoma.

**Breakout Point**

- Presents as burning epigastric pain
- *H. pylori* and NSAIDs are the most common causes
- Cannot turn into cancer

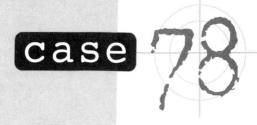

**ID/CC** A **42-year-old woman** is hospitalized with **fatigue, jaundice,** and **itching.**

**HPI** The patient is currently being treated for rheumatoid arthritis.

**PE** VS: normal. PE: **jaundice;** scleral icterus; **hepatomegaly** and hepatic tenderness; **xanthomas** on elbows and knees; skin hyperpigmentation.

**Labs** Hypercholesterolemia (>200 mg/dL). LFTs: **elevated alkaline phosphatase;** elevated bilirubin. **Positive antimitochondrial antibodies;** increased IgM levels.

**Imaging** ERCP: markedly decreased arborization of the intrahepatic biliary tree; the extrahepatic biliary tree appears normal in this patient.

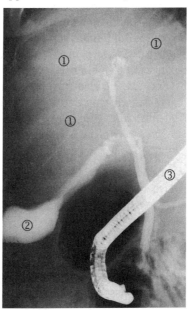

**Figure 78-1.** ERCP: markedly decreased arborization (*1*) of the intrahepatic biliary tree; the extrahepatic biliary tree appears normal in this patient. Note the gallbladder (*2*) and endoscope (*3*).

# case 78

## Primary Biliary Cirrhosis

**Pathogenesis**

Primary biliary cirrhosis is an idiopathic **autoimmune disease** characterized by the presence of **anti-mito-chondrial antibodies** and by the **destruction and loss of interlobular bile ducts,** leading to **severe obstructive jaundice** and **hypercholesterolemia.** Impaired bile excretion may result in malabsorption of fat-soluble vitamins (vitamins A, D, E, and K). The disease progresses to hepatic cirrhosis, portal hypertension, and complications arising from these conditions.

**Epidemiology**

Almost all symptomatic cases occur in **women aged 35 to 60 years.**

**Management**

Symptomatic treatment of pruritus may be achieved with cholestyramine or colestipol. Treatment of hyperlipidemia may require chronic **dietary modification** and use of **lipid-lowering drugs.** Agents include resins (e.g., cholestyramine), statins (e.g., lovastatin), and niacin. Gemfibrozil is indicated if hyperlipidemia includes elevated triglycerides. In primary biliary cirrhosis, the typical treatment is **ursodeoxycholic acid,** which delays the progression of the disease. Currently, **liver transplant** is the only definitive therapy.

**Complications**

Liver failure; steatorrhea; renal tubular acidosis; increased risk of hepatobiliary malignancies; fat-soluble vitamin deficiency states; increased cardiovascular risk (from hypercholesterolemia).

**Breakout Point**

- Presents as painless jaundice and pruritus in females
- Anti-mitochondrial antibodies
- Liver transplant is the only definitive therapy
- Associated with other autoimmune diseases

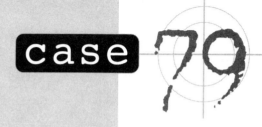

**ID/CC**  A **35-year-old woman** presents with **bloody diarrhea**, lower abdominal cramping pain, and associated tenesmus; she also reports significant **weight loss, fatigue, and light-headedness.**

**HPI**  She has suffered similar episodes in the past that have been treated as bacillary dysentery. Her grandmother suffered from inflammatory bowel disease.

**PE**  VS: low-grade fever (38.1°C); tachycardia (HR 110); orthostatic hypotension. PE: pallor; mild tenderness in lower abdomen; heme-positive brown stool.

**Labs**  CBC: normochromic, normocytic anemia; mild leukocytosis (13,000). Low serum albumin; colonoscopy shows diffuse, **continuous rectal involvement and friable fiery red mucosal areas;** rectal biopsy shows **superficial inflammation with crypt abscesses;** stool cultures negative; stool ova and parasites negative; P-ANCA positive.

**Imaging**  See Figure 79-1.

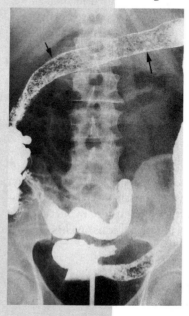

**Figure 79-1.** BE (avoid during acute phase). Loss of haustral markings; narrow, foreshortened colon and loss of redundancy in the rectosigmoid region (LEAD PIPE COLON) (*arrows*); microulcerations.

GI

# case 79

## Ulcerative Colitis

**Pathogenesis**

Ulcerative colitis is primarily an inflammatory disease affecting the superficial epithelial layer of the rectum and the colon. Disease begins in the rectum and progresses proximally in a continuous fashion (no skip lesions) to involve the colon; remissions and exacerbations are common. The etiology of this disease is unknown; chronic inflammation suggests that the cause may be a regulatory alteration of mucosal immunity.

**Epidemiology**

Ulcerative occurs more frequently in **whites** and affects 30% more **females** than males. It is two to four times more common among **Jews** than among non-Jews. Ten percent of patients have **family members** within two generations who also have the disease, and more than one-third know of a relative who has it. Incidence of ulcerative colitis peaks between 15 to 25 years of age and 55 to 65 years of age.

**Management**

**Bowel rest** and IV fluids; drugs used include antibiotics (cipro/flagyl), 5-ASA derivatives, **corticosteroids** (systemic or enemas), or immunosuppressive agents such as infliximab and azathioprine in severe cases that are refractory to corticosteroids. **Surgery** is indicated in refractory disease, toxic megacolon, colon cancer, and severe dysplasia. Perform **surveillance colonoscopy** annually after 8 to 10 years of disease; consider prophylactic colectomy in view of the markedly increased risk of colon cancer.

**Complications**

Complications include **toxic megacolon**, intestinal perforation, severe bleeding, and increased risk of **colon cancer**. Extraintestinal manifestations include **ankylosing spondylitis, erythema nodosum, pyoderma gangrenosum**, aphthous ulcers, and **iritis/uveitis**.

**Breakout Point**

- Presents as crampy bloody diarrhea
- Continuous red inflamed colonic mucosa
- Associated with extraintestinal manifestations
- Increased incidence of colon malignancy

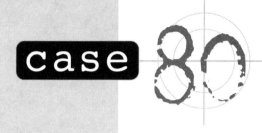

## case 80

| | |
|---|---|
| **ID/CC** | A **19-year-old woman** presents with **tremor, ataxia,** and **dysarthria.** |
| **HPI** | Her symptoms have gotten progressively worse over several months. Her family notes that her **personality** has **changed** and that she has been acting bizarrely. |
| **PE** | VS: normal. PE: slightly **jaundiced** female; slit lamp exam shows a greenish-gold pigment deposition in the corneal limbus **(Kayser–Fleischer ring)**; abdomen is soft with mild right upper quadrant tenderness and hepatomegaly; neurologic exam demonstrates an asymmetric tremor, **ataxic gait, increased muscle tone,** and dysarthric speech. |
| **Labs** | CBC, Chem7: normal. LFT: moderately elevated. **Low serum ceruloplasmin** (<20 mg/dL). Urine and CSF copper levels are elevated. |
| **Imaging** | Brain MRI: high signal intensity in the **basal ganglia** on T2-weighted images. Liver biopsy: fatty infiltrate in hepatocytes and portal fibrosis. Copper staining shows elevated copper levels. |

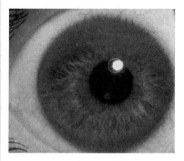

**Figure 80-1.** Kayser–Fleischer ring (greenish gold pigment deposition at the corneal limbus).

# case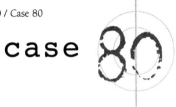

## Wilson Disease

**Pathogenesis**

Wilson disease (also called **hepatolenticular degeneration**) is an autosomal recessive disorder due to dysfunctional copper metabolism by the liver. The liver is unable to excrete copper into bile and has a limited ability to incorporate copper into ceruloplasmin. Copper builds up in the liver and causes hepatic destruction by releasing free radicals. Eventually copper spills into the serum and builds up in tissues of the **brain, kidneys, and eyes.** Children and adolescents initially present with symptoms of **liver dysfunction.** Older children and young adults present with **neuropsychiatric symptoms.** Damage to the **basal ganglia** can lead to **Parkinsonian-like** tremors, rigidity, and dystonia. Copper accumulation in the brain can also cause psychosis, mania, bizarre behavior, depression, and personality changes. Kidney dysfunction can present as nephrolithiasis or *Fanconi syndrome.* Copper deposition in the eyes results in **Kayser–Fleischer rings.**

**Epidemiology**

Wilson disease is a rare **autosomal recessive** disorder of copper metabolism. The genetic defect is localized to **chromosome 13.** The incidence is 1 per 30,000 people. Diagnosis is usually made between the **ages of 6 and 20.**

**Management**

The mainstay of therapy is treatment with copper **chelating agents. Zinc** is used to help bind copper in the intestine and prevent its absorption. Patients should eat a **low-copper diet,** avoiding foods such as nuts, chocolate, shellfish, and mushrooms.
Advanced disease may require liver transplant.

**Complications**

Presents as neuropsychiatric disturbance and liver dysfunction in a young adult.

**Breakout Point**

- Autosomal recessive
- Hepatolenticular degeneration
- Decreased ceruloplasmin

# questions

1. A 33-year-old woman presents to the emergency room complaining of fatigue and shortness of breath. For the last 2 weeks, she has noticed that she has very little energy and gets winded by walking up a flight of stairs. She was able to continue working until yesterday when she developed a fever of 102°F and a productive cough. Today her gums began to bleed when she was brushing her teeth. She denies any recent travel and does not know of any sick contacts. Physical exam was essentially unremarkable except for scattered petechiae. CBC reveals a WBC of 25,000, a hematocrit of 19, and a platelet count of 45. The differential on her white blood cell count showed 25% blasts. Her INR was 1.6, fibrinogen was 100, Cr was 1.8, and uric acid was 12. What is the most likely diagnosis?

   A. Acute myelogenous leukemia (AML)
   B. Chronic myelogenous leukemia (CML)
   C. Chronic lymphocytic leukemia (CLL)
   D. Acute lymphoblastic leukemia (ALL)
   E. Lymphoma

2. A 58-year-old African-American woman with a past medical history of temporal arteritis presents to your office for her annual visit. CBC reveals WBC of 12.3, Hb of 11.0, Hct of 33.7, platelets of 423,000, and MCV of 82. Iron studies show iron of 23 (low), TIBC of 220 (low), transferrin of 215 (normal), ferritin of 680 (high), and reticulocyte count of 1.2% (normal). Peripheral smear showed microcytic, hypochromic red blood cells, with normal myeloid precursors and normal-appearing platelets. There was no evidence of schistocytes, spherocytes, or sickled cells on her smear. Her lab studies are most consistent with which type of anemia?

   A. Iron-deficiency anemia
   B. Anemia of chronic disease
   C. $B_{12}$ deficiency
   D. Anemia consistent with sickle-cell disease
   E. Hemolytic anemia

3. A 65-year-old man with a 40-pack-year history of tobacco use, hypertension, and hyperlipidemia presents with severe chest pain radiating to his back. Over the past year, he has also noted increasing chest pressure and shortness of breath with climbing two flights of stairs.

161

On physical examination, he has a blood pressure of 188/100, pulse of 120 beats per minute, and oxygen saturation of 96% on room air. Faint carotid bruits are heard bilaterally and upstrokes are normal. Heart sounds are normal without murmurs, rubs, or gallops. Lungs are clear to auscultation. An ECG shows T-wave inversions in leads V2-V6. Chest radiography shows a widened mediastinum with clear lungs. What is the most appropriate next step in the management of this patient?

A. Administration of sublingual nitroglycerin
B. Administration of aspirin
C. Chest CT with contrast
D. Chest MRI with contrast
E. Diagnostic coronary angiography

4. A 37-year-old woman with a history of diabetes, gastroesophageal reflux disease, and HIV presents with odynophagia for 2 weeks. Pain occurs just after she swallows and causes difficulty with eating solids and liquids. She has lost 5 pounds during this time period and has had subjective fevers. On physical exam, her temperature is 100.4°F, blood pressure is 110/80, heart rate is 95, and oxygen saturation is 97% on room air. She has a white coating on her tongue and her buccal mucosa. Upper endoscopy demonstrates white plaques along the lining of the esophagus. Brush biopsy shows yeasts and pseudo-hyphae invading mucosal cells. Which of the following statements is true about her disease?

A. This is not an AIDS-defining illness.
B. The white coating and plaques are likely bacterial exudates.
C. All patients who have this esophageal disease will have oral lesions as well.
D. Predisposing factors for development of this disease include use of antibiotics, chemotherapy, or inhaled corticosteroids.
E. These lesions can progress to cancer.

5. A 30-year-old woman presents to your office with complaints of 3 days of throat, jaw, and ear pain. In addition, she complains of fatigue and myalgias. She notes that she had an upper respiratory infection 2 weeks prior consisting of rhinorrhea and cough, but these symptoms have since resolved. Her temperature is 100.1°F, pulse is 103, blood pressure is 130/80, and respiratory rate is 13. Her tympanic membranes are clear, her oropharynx is nonerythematous, and she has no tem-poromandibular joint tenderness. She has no subdmandibular or cervical lymphadenopathy. The thyroid gland is moderately enlarged on examination with marked left-sided thyroid gland tenderness.

Laboratory values reveal a white blood cell count of 13.0, a hematocrit of 34.0, an undetectable TSH level, and a free T4 level elevated at 15. Radioiodine uptake scan reveals no uptake. Which of the following is true about this patient's diagnosis?

A. Thyroid autoimmunity plays a primary role in the pathogenesis of this disorder.

B. Most patients will have a high titer of serum antiperoxidase or antithyroglobulin antibodies.

C. A thionamide such as methimazole would be a reasonable component of therapy.

D. A reasonable initial therapy would be initiation of prednisone.

E. An erythrocyte sedimentation rate (ESR) of 90 would not be consistent with this diagnosis.

6. A 45-year-old African-American male is brought to the emergency room after being found wandering aimlessly on the street in a disoriented state. The patient appears to be confused and agitated. His wife reports that the patient was diagnosed with essential hypertension 3 weeks ago and was started on hydrochlorothiazide. He has not been compliant with the regimen due to problems with impotence. Per report, the patient also has a history of cocaine use. On examination, the patient is afebrile with blood pressure of 220/130, equal in both arms, heart rate of 110 beats per minute, respiration rate of 20/min, and an $O_2$ saturation of 98% on room air. The patient is agitated, diaphoretic, with dilated but reactive pupils. He vomits in the emergency room. Fundoscopic exam reveals papilledema and scattered retinal hemorrhages. His heart, lung, and abdominal examinations are normal. The pulses are strong and equal in arms and legs. He is able to follow commands but is slightly tremulous. Basic metabolic panel and complete blood count are normal. CT scan of the head is negative for acute hemorrhage. Due to persistent neurological symptoms, an MRI of the head is also obtained and shows no acute infarction or hemorrhage, but T2-weighted images reveal edema of the white matter of the parieto-occipital regions. Urine toxin screen is negative for cocaine metabolites. What is the best strategy for initial management?

A. Start treatment for cocaine withdrawal.

B. Lower the diastolic pressure to 100 to 105 mm Hg with the maximum initial fall not exceeding 25% of the presenting value.

C. Restart previous outpatient dose of hydrochlorothiazide.

D. Immediately lower blood pressure to 120/80 with intravenous medications.

E. Recheck blood pressure as an outpatient.

7. A thin 50-year-old woman has had progressive fatigue, dyspnea on exertion, and palpitations over the past year. On physical examination, her blood pressure is 148/40 with a pulse of 85. Carotid upstrokes are rapid. The cardiac apical impulse is diffuse and displaced laterally. Cardiac auscultation reveals an absent S2 and soft murmur that decreases in intensity from S2 to S1. The murmur increases with squatting and decreases with valsalva maneuvers. Chest radiography shows cardiomegaly and a widened mediastinum. Which of the following is correct?

   A. The intensity of her murmur signifies a poor prognosis.
   B. Her condition is associated with inflammatory bowel disease.
   C. A congenital malformation of the valve is an uncommon etiology for the symptoms.
   D. She is at high risk for the development of ventricular arrhythmias.
   E. She does not need antibiotic prophylaxis for endocarditis.

8. A 76-year-old man with a past medical history of diabetes and hypertension presents to the emergency department with a single episode of transient left upper extremity weakness. It lasted approximately 45 minutes and resolved completely. He denies having any prior similar events. He reports intermittent sensation of palpitations over the last year. Physical exam reveals an elderly appearing man in no apparent distress with a blood pressure of 150/90, pulse 126, respiratory rate 16, and temperature 97.5°F. On auscultation, his heart sounds are irregular and no murmurs are appreciated. Lungs are clear to auscultation bilaterally and there is no lower extremity edema. His neurologic exam is nonfocal. CT head reveals no evidence of bleeding. His ECG shows absence of P-waves and an irregular rhythm with a ventricular rate of 126. A transthoracic echocardiogram was obtained revealing a left ventricular ejection fraction of 30% and left ventricular hypertrophy, with no significant valvular abnormalities. Which of the following is true about his condition?

   A. The patient should be converted to normal sinus rhythm with medications due to his high risk for cardioembolic disease.
   B. This patient should be immediately cardioverted.
   C. The findings on echocardiogram are associated with a higher thromboembolic risk.
   D. This patient will have to be on lifelong anticoagulation with a target INR of 3.0 to 4.0.
   E. Digoxin is generally considered first-line therapy.

9. A 65-year-old man with a history of COPD, CAD, status post-CABG 1 month ago, presents to the emergency room complaining of feeling faint, light-headed, and nauseous. On further questioning, the patient also reports "irregular heartbeat" and chest tightness over the past 2 weeks. He has also become increasingly dyspneic, especially on exertion, but has attributed this problem to a recent "chest cold" he has been going through. This past week, he has increased his use of his albuterol inhaler to 2 puffs every 2 hours without significant relief of his symptoms. Physical examination revealed a pale elderly gentleman in mild respiratory distress. Temperature is 101.0°F, heart exam revealed rapid, irregular heartbeat of 160 beats per minute. Blood pressure was 100/60. Respiratory rate was at 20 breaths per minute and labored, and oxygen saturation is 89% on room air. Other significant findings included perioral cyanosis and clubbing of the fingernails. ECG reveals a narrow-complex, irregular rhythm at the rate of around 120 bpm with at least three different P-wave morphologies in a single lead (II). What is the most likely rhythm?

A. Atrial fibrillation
B. Atrial flutter
C. Multifocal atrial tachycardia
D. Regular sinus tachycardia
E. Normal sinus rhythm

10. A 39-year-old Caucasian woman with a history of hypertension presents to the emergency department with severe right upper quadrant pain and abdominal distension for the past week. She reports regular alcohol use and reports smoking $\frac{1}{2}$ pack per day × 10 years. Her only medication is an oral contraceptive. On exam, she is noted to have a low-grade temperature, scleral icterus, and jaundice. Her abdomen is distended with shifting dullness noted and tenderness to palpation of the RUQ quadrant. Murphy sign is negative. The liver edge is approximated at 4 cm below the costal margin. An abdominal ultrasound with Doppler reveals an occlusive thrombus in the right hepatic vein. Which aspect of the patient's history is most likely to be the cause for her presentation?

A. Gender of the patient
B. History of hypertension
C. Ethnicity of the patient
D. Oral contraceptive use
E. Regular alcohol intake

11. A 28-year-old man presents to the office with complaints of chronic diarrhea. He has had persistent, bulky diarrhea with a foul odor for 3 months. This has been associated with abdominal bloating, increased flatulence, and fatigue. He has developed restless legs and fissuring at the corners of his mouth. He also describes a waxing and waning itchy rash consisting of grouped vesicles on his elbows and buttocks. He has not been camping or traveling recently and has no sick contacts. Physical exam shows a tired, pale-appearing male with angular cheilosis. He has mild tenderness on abdominal exam. He has grouped vesicles over the elbows and buttocks, some of which are excoriated. Diagnostic studies demonstrate a hemoglobin of 10.0 with an MCV of 75 and slightly prolonged PTT. His tissue transglutaminase antibody is found to be positive, and he is set up for an endoscopy and small bowel biopsy. Which of the following is true about this disease?

    A. Small bowel biopsy will classically show villous atrophy.
    B. Discontinuing intake of dairy products will likely resolve his symptoms.
    C. He has symptoms consistent with vitamin $B_1$ deficiency due to decreased small bowel absorption.
    D. This disease is prevalent in the Asian population.
    E. His skin lesions represent pyoderma gangrenosum, which is commonly associated with this disease.

12. A 60-year-old man with a past medical history of hypertension, type II diabetes mellitus, and tobacco abuse presents to your office with a chief complaint of weight loss. He has had a poor appetite over the last few months and is losing weight. However, he notes that when he does eat, he feels like he gets full quickly. He also complains of generalized fatigue and malaise. Physical exam is only notable for a mildly enlarged spleen. A CBC reveals a WBC of 167,000 with a differential showing 30 neutrophils, 23 lymphocytes, 16 metamyelocytes, 14 myelocytes, 7 promyelocytes, 4 blasts, 2 eosinophils, and 4 basophils. His hematocrit is low at 35 and his platelet count is elevated at 575,000. Nucleated red blood cells were also seen on the smear. What mutation is the most likely cause of his disease?

    A. t(15;17)
    B. t(9;22)
    C. t(8;21)
    D. inv16
    E. 11q23

13. A 45-year-old woman with a past medical history of hypertension and hyperlipidemia presents for a routine checkup. She denies any current complaints or symptoms, but reports that she has had frequent yeast infections over the past 6 months. Physical exam reveals an obese female with a BP of 130/90 and HR of 70. Pelvic exam is unremarkable. Routine labs are drawn at the visit, including a fasting serum glucose, which returns at 160 mg/dL. What is the appropriate next step in management?

    A. Start the patient on insulin therapy.
    B. Have the patient return for a repeat fasting plasma glucose.
    C. Check a glycosylated hemoglobin level.
    D. Recommend the patient cut down her sugar intake.
    E. Begin the patient on metformin.

14. A 68-year-old man with a history of diabetes and hypertension presents for his annual physical exam. For the past several months, he reports increased fatigue. His physical exam is within normal limits. Labs are notable for a WBC of 40 with a lymphocytic predominance. Peripheral smear is significant for "smudge cells." Which of the following is characteristic of this disease?

    A. Treatment can be curative if initiated early before symptoms occur.
    B. This is a rapidly progressive disease.
    C. Patients can develop refractory immune thrombocytopenia.
    D. The majority of cases will progress to a diffuse large cell lymphoma known as Richter syndrome.
    E. The median survival time is 1 year.

15. A 30-year-old woman with HIV presents to the ED with confusion, generalized malaise, vomiting, and diarrhea for the past 3 days. Her vitals are: T 101, BP 100/80, HR 100, R24, $O_2$sat 95% on 2L by nasal cannula. Physical examination is noteworthy for an ill-appearing female with dry mucous membranes and scattered petechiae on her shins. Her urine output for the past 8 hours has been 200 mL. Labs are significant for a Hct of 26 (baseline 32), elevated reticulocyte count, platelet count of 80, and Cr of 2.0 (baseline 1.0). Which of the following statements is true about this condition?

    A. It is a consumptive coagulopathy without involvement of the kidneys and CNS.
    B. Even without treatment, renal failure is usually reversible.
    C. It is associated with oral contraceptive use and pregnancy.
    D. Treatment is not started until the patient is symptomatic.
    E. Characteristic lab findings include increased fibrin split products, decreased fibrinogen, and increased d-dimer.

16. A 50-year-old man with a history of peptic ulcer disease presents with a complaint of persistent epigastric pain, worsened with spicy foods. He takes a proton-pump inhibitor for his peptic ulcer disease but continues to have symptoms of epigastric pain, heartburn with meals, and frequent diarrhea. His last EGD was several years ago and demonstrated multiple ulcers in the duodenum and jejunum. *Helicobacter pylori* serology was negative at that time. He was referred to a gastroenterologist who performs a repeat EGD. The repeat endoscopy showed the same ulcers that have failed to heal despite therapy. What is the next best step in determining the etiology of the patient's symptoms?

    A. Serum gastrin levels
    B. CT scan of the abdomen
    C. Ultrasound of the abdomen
    D. Secretin stimulation test
    E. MRI of the abdomen

17. A 50-year-old man presents for a routine primary care visit. He has been having mild abdominal discomfort, but otherwise has been feeling well. Laboratory testing shows a serum calcium of 11.0 mg/dL (elevated), serum parathyroid hormone of 142 ng/L (elevated), normal CBC, and normal LFTs. A 24-hour urinary calcium is 272 mg, and alkaline phosphatase is normal. The patient is found to have primary hyperparathyroidism. Which of the following is true of this condition?

    A. It is most commonly caused by parathyroid carcinoma.
    B. Patients are usually very symptomatic on initial presentation.
    C. Prognosis is poor for this patient due to severity of complications.
    D. Parathyroidectomy should be performed immediately for this patient.
    E. The most common cause is parathyroid adenoma.

18. A 55-year-old man presents with several-month history of weakness and fatigue. He reports a 15-pound unintentional weight loss. Recently he has noticed bleeding from his gums and small red spots on his skin. Physical exam is noteworthy for conjunctival pallor, scattered petechiae, and hepatosplenomegaly. Labs are significant for an elevated WBC of 30 with a blast predominance. Which of the following is true of this disease?

A. Treatment includes surgery to remove excess bone marrow.
B. It has a bimodal age distribution, occurring most commonly in children and later in adults older than age 50.
C. Philadelphia chromosome (translocation 9:22) carries a good prognosis.
D. Very few adults go into complete remission after therapy.
E. It is a disease of older adults characterized by circulating mature lymphocytes.

19. A 40-year-old woman with a history of hepatitis C and cirrhosis is admitted with a several-month history of abdominal pain, weight loss, and fatigue. Despite decreased oral intake, she notes increased abdominal girth. She denies any nausea, vomiting, fevers, or chills. Vital signs are within normal limits. On physical exam her liver is palpable 2 cm below the R costal margin. There is no rebound tenderness or guarding. A CT of the abdomen shows an enhancing liver mass measuring approximately 3 cm. Labs are significant for decreased serum albumin, elevated LFTs, elevated PT, and AFP is >400 μg/L. Which of the following is true of this condition?

    A. It is most commonly associated with viral infections.
    B. The degree of LFT elevation correlates with degree of progression.
    C. Elevated AFP is a sign of good prognosis.
    D. There are no therapy options for this condition.
    E. Liver biopsy is not performed because of risk of bleeding.

20. A 30-year-old man presents to your clinic to establish primary care. For the past several months he has been feeling very tired and bruises easily. His recent teeth cleaning was complicated by mucosal bleeding. Physical exam is notable for moderate splenomegaly. Lab studies are significant for a platelet count of 1,000,000. Blood smear shows hypogranular megakaryocytes. Which of the following is characteristic of this disease?

    A. It tends to arise from inflammation, iron deficiency, or acute bleeding.
    B. It is caused by Epstein–Barr virus infection.
    C. Patients with elevated platelet counts may experience transient ischemic attacks.
    D. Associated splenomegaly is rare.
    E. Most patients progress to an aggressive form of leukemia.

# answers

**1-A**

A. Acute myeloid leukemia [Correct] can occur at any age, but the incidence tends to increase with age. It often presents acutely and the most common presenting symptom is fatigue, due to the profound anemia these patients often experience. On presentation, patients may also have infections due to impaired neutrophil function. Bleeding can also be present, due to either thrombocytopenia or DIC, depending on what type of AML is present. The diagnosis can be made by the presence of >20% blasts in the peripheral blood or bone marrow.

B. Chronic myelogenous leukemia [Incorrect] usually occurs in patients aged 40 to 60. Laboratory evaluation will often reveal a markedly elevated WBC and there will be evidence of all myeloid precursors on peripheral smear. The number of blasts is usually low, unless the patient has advanced through the stages of CML and is now in blast crisis, progressing to an acute leukemia.

C. Chronic lymphocytic leukemia [Incorrect] primarily affects adults >65 years old and is considered a chronic, indolent disease. It is often asymptomatic for many years and diagnosed simply by finding an elevated WBC on routine bloodwork. Other blood counts are usually normal. Smudge cells on a peripheral smear are diagnostic.

D. Acute lymphocytic leukemia [Incorrect] occurs most often in children, but can occur in adults. It can be of either B- or T- cell origin. The prognosis is better in children than in adults.

E. Lymphoma [Incorrect] often presents with "B symptoms" of fevers, night sweats, and weight loss. On physical exam, patients often have lymphadenopathy.

**2-B**

A. In pure iron-deficiency anemia [Incorrect], findings would include a low iron, high TIBC, and a low ferritin.

B. Anemia of chronic disease [Correct] is typified by any level of serum iron, low TIBC, and high ferritin. This type of anemia presents in conjunction with a chronic inflammatory condition (such as temporal arteritis).

C. $B_{12}$ deficiency [Incorrect] results in a macrocytic anemia, typically with an MCV >100 (not 82).

D. In anemia consistent with sickle-cell disease [Incorrect], sickle cells would likely be visible on the peripheral smear. The MCV would also be low and her anemia would likely be much worse.

E. Hemolytic anemia [Incorrect] causes schistocytes on the peripheral smear. Other lab abnormalities associated with hemolytic anemia include a decreased haptoglobin, elevated LDH, elevated reticulocyte count, and elevated total bilirubin.

**3-C**

A. Sublingual nitroglycerin [Incorrect] is administered for suspicion of acute coronary syndrome; in dissection, intravenous metoprolol would be most appropriate for decreasing significantly elevated blood pressure. If this were a descending aorta dissection, long-term therapy with oral beta-blockers would be appropriate, but the type of dissection cannot be determined without imaging.

B. Aspirin [Incorrect] should be avoided in the acute setting since it would make control of any bleeding more difficult.

C. This patient has an aortic dissection. The type of dissection is not clear until rapid imaging such as CT chest [Correct] is performed to evaluate the extent and need for immediate surgery versus medical management.

D. MRI of chest [Incorrect] would give excellent resolution of the dissection, but is time-consuming and not the first test of choice.

E. Diagnostic coronary angiography [Incorrect] is performed in cases of high suspicion for acute coronary ischemia. If the dissection extended into the coronary arteries, ST-segment elevations on electrocardiography would be expected.

**4-D**

A. Esophageal candidiasis is an AIDS-defining illness [Incorrect] that occurs in patients with HIV with a CD4 count <200.

B. The white coating on her oral mucosa and plaques [Incorrect] in her esophagus are most commonly caused by *Candida albicans,* not bacteria.

C. The absence of oral thrush [Incorrect] does not exclude a patient from having esophageal candidiasis. Patients may present with isolated esophageal infection without oral lesions.

D. This patient has esophageal candidiasis. Predisposing factors include HIV, immunosuppressive agents, antibiotic use [Correct], diabetes mellitus, and esophageal motility disorders.

E. These lesions do not progress to cancer [Incorrect]; complications of esophageal candidiasis are rare and can include ulceration, bleeding, fistula formation, and fibrosis.

**5-D**

A. Thyroid autoimmunity [Incorrect] is not the primary cause in pathogenesis, although inflammatory cell infiltration of the thyroid does occur. Thyroid autoimmunity plays a classic role in the pathogenesis of Graves disease and Hashimoto thyroiditis.

B. A high serum titer of serum antiperoxidase or antithyroglobulin antibodies [Incorrect] is not found in De Quervain thyroiditis, but instead is found in Hashimoto thyroiditis and Graves disease.

C. Methimazole [Incorrect] is not used to treat De Quervain thyroiditis, since this condition is not caused by excess thyroid hormone synthesis. Initial management is an anti-inflammatory regimen such as NSAIDs; corticosteroids may be used in refractory cases.

D. This case describes DeQuervain thyroiditis (also called subacute granulomatous thyroiditis), for which a reasonable initial therapy is prednisone [Correct].

E. An elevated ESR over 50 [Incorrect] and at times over 100 (is typical of DeQuervain thyroiditis.

**6-B**

A. Cocaine (or stimulant) withdrawal syndrome [Incorrect] is characterized by a drastic reduction in mood and energy that starts 15 to 30 minutes after cessation of a stimulant binge. High blood pressure and delirium usually do not occur.

B. Hypertensive emergency is defined as an episode of elevated blood pressure associated with acute end-organ damage or dysfunction and requires carefully controlled lowering of blood pressure in an inpatient setting. Hypertensive urgency, on the other hand, is defined as an episode of elevated blood pressure without associated acute end-organ damage, and patients can usually be started back on an oral regimen and reassessed as an outpatient in 24 to 48 hours. In this case, the patient's neurologic symptoms (confusion, agitation, disorientation) are indicative of end-organ damage, such as that seen in hypertensive encephalopathy. The MRI findings of edema of the white matter of the parieto-occipital regions, termed reversible posterior leukoencephalopathy syndrome, occurs with malignant hypertension. The initial management for hypertensive emergency should consist of admission to the intensive care unit, and gently lowering the diastolic pressure to about 100 to 105 mm Hg with the maximum initial fall in blood pressure not exceeding 25% of the presenting value [Correct]. More aggressive hypotensive therapy may reduce the blood pressure below the autoregulatory range, possibly leading to ischemic events such as stroke and myocardial infarction.

C. Restarting the outpatient dose of hydrochlorothiazide [Incorrect] may be appropriate for certain cases of hypertensive urgency, but since this patient is experiencing end-organ damage from malignant hypertension (neurologic symptoms and MRI findings), more intensive therapy and observation are required.

D. Blood pressure should not be immediately lowered to 120/80 [Incorrect]. The blood pressure needs to be lowered gradually, by decreasing blood pressure by 25% in the first 2 to 6 hours.

E. Because of end-organ damage and severity of symptoms, it would not be appropriate to only recheck the blood pressure as an outpatient [Incorrect].

**7-B**

A. The intensity of the murmur [Incorrect] does not correlate with prognosis or progression of disease.

B. This patient has classic physical exam findings of aortic regurgitation (AR), with a wide pulse pressure, diastolic murmur, and evidence of cardiomegaly. AR may occur from a variety of disorders leading to abnormalities of the aortic valve or dilatation of the aortic root, including collagen vascular disease and inflammatory bowel disease [Correct].

C. One of the most common etiologies of AR is congenital bicuspid aortic valve [Incorrect], especially in developed countries.

D. Arrhythmias [Incorrect] are not a common complication of AR. Palpitations can be due to compensatory tachycardia or premature ventricular beats, but sustained arrhythmias are uncommon.

E. Antibiotic prophylaxis to prevent endocarditis [Incorrect] is recommended when a patient is at risk for bacteremia, including dental or invasive procedures. Patients with AR are considered to be at moderate risk for endocarditis by the American Heart Association.

**8-C**

A. The patient should not be converted to normal sinus rhythm [Incorrect] with medications or cardioversion at this time, for increased risk of embolism.

B. Immediate cardioversion [Incorrect] is the therapy of choice in hemodynamically unstable patients, but this patient has stable vital signs.

C. This patient has had a transient ischemic attack (TIA) causing transient left upper extremity weakness. His condition of atrial fibrillation predisposes him to TIA and cerebrovascular accident. The presence of a decreased left ventricular ejection fraction and left ventricular hypertrophy is associated with a higher thromboembolic risk. Transesophageal echocardiogram has been shown to identify features that correlate with high thromboembolic risk [Correct], such as left atrial thrombus, left atrial appendage size, left ventricular dysfunction, left ventricular hypertrophy, and complex aortic plaque.

D. The currently recommended target INR range [Incorrect] is 2.0 to 3.0 for prevention of stroke in atrial fibrillation. This patient is at high risk for stroke given his history of hypertension, diabetes, age >75, and clinical presentation consistent with a transient ischemic attack. Most strokes occur at an INR below 2.0. Likewise, most bleeding episodes tend to occur at an INR that exceeds 3.0.

E. Digoxin [Incorrect] is only effective for rate control at rest and therefore should only be used as a second-line agent for rate control. First-line agents for heart rate control in atrial fibrillation are beta-blockers and calcium-channel blockers.

**9-C**

A. Atrial fibrillation [Incorrect] is often confused with multifocal atrial tachycardia, due to a similar irregularly irregular rhythm and similar predisposing conditions, but in atrial fibrillation, no P-waves are seen on ECG.

B. The classic ECG finding in atrial flutter [Incorrect] is a saw-tooth pattern of waves.

C. This is a classic example of multifocal atrial tachycardia [Correct]. The term multifocal atrial tachycardia is used when atrial impulses show at least three different P-wave morphologies and the ventricular rate is 100 or greater. Multifocal atrial tachycardia is frequently associated with chronic obstructive lung disease, which this patient has.

D. Regular sinus tachycardia [Incorrect] is incorrect, since the rhythm is regular.

E. Normal sinus rhythm [Incorrect] is incorrect, since the rhythm is regular, and the rate in normal sinus rhythm should range from 60 to 100 (not 160).

**10-D**

A. Gender of the patient [Incorrect] does not play a causative role, since this syndrome affects both females and males equally.

B. Hypertension [Incorrect] does not predispose to thrombosis as is seen in Budd–Chiari, and it alone will not induce icterus or jaundice.

C. Ethnicity of the patient [Incorrect] is not relevant, since the development of Budd–Chiari has no racial predilection.

D. This patient is presenting with Budd–Chiari syndrome, which is defined as a process that results in the interruption of normal blood flow out of the liver. It commonly implies thrombosis of the inferior vena cava and/or major hepatic veins, as described in this case. Major causes of Budd–Chiari include malignancy, pregnancy, oral contraceptives [Correct], myeloproliferative disorders, hypercoaguable states, and infectious/benign lesions of the liver.

E. Regular alcohol intake [Incorrect] is not a predisposing factor to thrombosis seen in Budd–Chiari, although it is a predisposing factor to cirrhosis.

## 11-A

A. This patient has celiac sprue, also called gluten-sensitive enteropathy. While patients with celiac sprue may have a normal-appearing small intestine, the classic small bowel biopsy shows atrophic or absent villi [Correct], elongated crypts, and increased mucosal lymphocytes and plasma cells. Strict adherence to a gluten-free diet is usually curative and can result in regression of the disease. Grains such as wheat, barley, rye, and oats contain gluten.

B. Some patients with celiac disease may have a secondary lactose intolerance, but discontinuing dairy products alone [Incorrect] will not result in resolution of disease.

C. Vitamin $B_1$ (thiamine) deficiency [Incorrect] results in beriberi and Wernicke–Korsakoff syndrome; this patient's symptoms of a prolonged PTT are from vitamin K deficiency due to malabsorption, not from vitamin $B_1$ deficiency. His restless legs, pale skin, and microcytic anemia are due to iron deficiency. Cheilosis can be due to iron, vitamin $B_2$, or $B_{12}$ deficiency.

D. Celiac sprue is rare in Asians [Incorrect] and Africans and prevalent in Western Europeans.

E. Pyoderma gangrenosum [Incorrect] is more commonly associated with inflammatory bowel diseases. His skin lesions represent dermatitis herpetiformis, which is associated with celiac disease.

## 12-B

A. t(15;17) [Incorrect] is the PML-RAR alpha mutation associated with acute myelogenous leukemia (AML). This fusion protein puts the nuclear transcription factor RAR under the control of PML and causes suppression of gene transcription. This translocation is the target of the drug *all-trans* retinoic acid (ATRA), which acts on RAR alpha and allows the cells to continue through differentiation, relieving the transcriptional block.

B. This patient has chronic myelogenous leukemia (CML). CML usually occurs in patients aged 40 to 60, with markedly elevated WBC and elevated myeloid precursors on peripheral smear, as is demonstrated in this case. t(9;22) [Correct] is a reciprocal chromosomal translocation known as the Philadelphia chromosome, which creates a BCR-ABL fusion protein. This protein results in a constitutively active tyrosine kinase. This protein is the target of the drug imatinib mesylate (Gleevec), which functionally shuts off the tyrosine kinase.

C. t(8;21) [Incorrect] is one of most common mutations in AML and indicates a good prognosis for treatment response.

D. inv 16 [Incorrect] is another mutation associated with AML which also bodes a favorable prognosis for treatment response.

E. 11q23 [Incorrect] is a mutation commonly seen in patients with AML due to previous chemotherapy, particularly with topoisomerase inhibitors. It carries a poorer prognosis in terms of treatment response.

**13-B**

A. Insulin therapy [Incorrect] should not be initiated until a repeat fasting glucose is checked.

B. The patient is to return for a repeat fasting serum glucose [Correct]. The diagnosis of diabetes mellitus is suspected in this patient given the elevated fasting glucose ≥126 mg/dL, the patient's history of hypertension and hyperlipidemia, and history of frequent yeast infections. However, the criteria to make a formal diagnosis of diabetes mellitus include fasting plasma glucose ≥126 mg/dL on two separate occasions; random glucose ≥200 mg/dL + classic symptoms (polyphagia, polydipsia, polyuria, weight loss); or 2-hour postglucose load (75 g) plasma glucose ≥200 mg/dL and confirmed on repeat test.

C. Glycosylated hemoglobin (or hemoglobin A1C) [Incorrect] levels are not useful for the diagnosis of diabetes mellitus because they are not standardized internationally and are insensitive to detecting milder forms of the disease. Hemoglobin A1C measurements are used to monitor long-term glycemic control and reflect glycemic control for the previous 3 months.

D. It is important that the patient is counseled about decreasing sugar intake [Incorrect], but lifestyle dietary modifications will likely not be sufficient in this case.

E. Metformin [Incorrect] should not be started; the diagnosis of diabetes mellitus should be confirmed prior to initiating any therapy.

**14-A**

A. Chronic lymphocytic leukemia (CLL) is characterized by a prolonged asymptomatic phase. Current treatment options are not curative [Correct], thus treatment is not initiatied until patients are symptomatic with fevers, evidence of bone marrow suppression, severe fatigue, or night sweats.

B. CLL is classically an indolent disease that may be incidentally uncovered; it is not a rapidly progressive disease [Incorrect].

C. Patients can develop refractory immune thrombocytopenia [Incorrect], which can be treated with steroids, intravenous immunoglobulin, or splenectomy.

D. Only 5% of cases will transform into a diffuse large B-cell lymphoma known as Richter syndrome, not the majority of cases [Incorrect].

E. The median survival time is 5 to 6 years, not 1 year [Incorrect].

**15-C**

A. TTP-HUS is a consumptive coagulopathy [Incorrect] characterized by mental status changes, renal failure, anemia, fever, and thrombocytopenia.

B. Renal failure is usually irreversible if treatment is not initiated [Incorrect]. Plasmapheresis, steroids, and supportive care are the mainstays of treatment.

C. This patient's presentation is consistent with thrombotic thrombocytopenic purpura-hemolytic uremic syndrome (TTP-HUS). TTP-HUS is associated with hypercoagulable tendency, as with oral contraceptive use and pregnancy [Correct].

D. Treatment should be initiated immediately if the diagnosis is suspected [Incorrect] because of the severity of sequelae; therapy should not be delayed until after the patient is symptomatic.

E. TTP-HUS can be distinguished from other microangiopathic disorders in that thrombocytopenia usually occurs without disseminated intravascular coagulation. Lab findings of increased fibrin split products, decreased fibrinogen, and increased d-dimer [Incorrect] are characteristic of DIC.

**16-A**

    A. This case describes Zollinger–Ellison syndrome. Diagnostic factors include atypical location of the ulcers (jejunum), ulcer disease in association with diarrhea, and ulcers that have failed to respond to medical therapy. The best screening test is a fasting serum gastrin level [Correct]; levels >1000 pg/mL are consistent with Zollinger–Ellison syndrome.

    B. CT abdomen [Incorrect] may be performed to localize the tumor once the diagnosis of Zollinger–Ellison is made, but is not the initial step in diagnosis.

    C. Ultrasound abdomen [Incorrect] is useful in conditions such as cholelithiasis, but it may not demarcate the tumor in Zollinger–Ellison.

    D. The secretin stimulation test [Incorrect] is a provocative test in which secretin is administered and serum levels of gastrin are determined at certain time points. This test is generally performed once initial serum gastrin levels are determined.

    E. MRI abdomen [Incorrect] is an imaging modality that can be used to localize the tumor of Zollinger–Ellison, but of note, CT scans are usually more sensitive than MRI or ultrasound in detecting these tumors.

**17-E**

    A. Parathyroid carcinoma [Incorrect] occurs in 2% of cases.

    B. Patients are typically asymptomatic on initial presentation [Incorrect], and elevated calcium is usually an incidental laboratory finding. Patients who are symptomatic manifest with arthralgias, abdominal discomfort, and nephrolithiasis.

    C. Prognosis is generally considered to be good [Incorrect] in primary hyperparathyroidism.

    D. Parathyroidectomy also does not have to immediately be performed [Incorrect]. Most asymptomatic patients who take a watchful waiting approach do not have a progression in their disease.

    E. Primary hyperparathyroidism is caused by an overproduction of parathyroid hormone. 80% of cases are caused by one or more parathyroid adenomas [Correct]. Parathyroid adenomas can be resected during parathyroidectomy.

**18-B**

    A. Treatment includes chemotherapy, radiation, and stem cell transplant, not surgery [Incorrect].

    B. This patient has acute lymphoblastic leukemia (ALL). ALL has a bimodal age distribution, occurring most commonly in children and later in adults older than age 50 [Correct].

C. Presence of the Philadelphia chromosome (translocation 9:22) [Incorrect] carries a poor prognosis in ALL.

D. The majority of adults [Incorrect], about 60% to 80%, go into complete remission (defined as <5% blasts) after induction therapy.

E. ALL can occur in older adults [Incorrect], but it is characterized by the presence of circulating lymphoblasts, not mature lymphocytes.

**19-A**

A. This patient has hepatocellular carcinoma (HCC). HCC is a neoplasm most commonly associated with viral infections [Correct] such as hepatitis B (Asia) or hepatitis C (United States). Patients with cirrhosis are also at an increased risk for HCC and should be monitored on a regular basis.

B. The degree of LFT elevation [Incorrect] may be variable and does not necessarily correlate with the degree of HCC progression. Long-term cirrhosis with a "burned-out" liver may actually result in normal LFT findings.

C. AFP [Incorrect] can be elevated in up to 50% of patients with HCC and is thus helpful in diagnosis, but is not an indicator of prognosis.

D. Therapy options for HCC [Incorrect] include initial evaluation with CT abdomen, followed by tumor embolization, chemotherapy, and/or surgical resection.

E. To confirm the diagnosis of HCC, a liver biopsy [Incorrect] is needed.

**20-C**

A. The etiology of essential thrombocytosis is unknown. Secondary thrombocytosis arises from known causes, such as inflammation, iron deficiency, or acute bleeding [Incorrect].

B. Infectious mononucleosis, an unrelated condition, is caused by Epstein–Barr virus infection [Incorrect].

C. This patient has essential thrombocytosis, in which patients may present with spontaneous bleeding, or arterial or venous thrombosis. Patients with elevated platelet counts may experience transient ischemic attacks [Correct].

D. Up to two-thirds of patients present with modest splenomegaly, thus associated splenomegaly is not rare [Incorrect].

E. A small percentage of cases [Incorrect] will progress to an aggressive form of leukemia, but this is an uncommon phenomenon.

# credits

Austen KF. *Samnter's Immunological Diseases.* 6th ed. Philadelphia: Lippincott Williams & Wilkins; 2003. Table 58-1 (Table 54-1).

Becker KL, Bilezikian JP, Brenner WJ, et al. *Principles and Practice of Endocrinology and Metabolism.* 3rd ed. Philadelphia: Lippincott Williams & Wilkins; 2001. Figs. 46-3 (30-1), 60-1 (33-1), 218-7A&B (34-1).

Bhushan V, Le T, Pall V. *Underground Clinical Vignettes: Step 2 Internal Medicine I.* 3rd ed. Malden, MA: Blackwell; 2005. Figs. 02 (2-1), 03 (3-1), 04 (4-1), 05A (6-1), 05B (6-2), 05C (6-3), 06A (7-1), 06B (7-2), 07 (8-1), 10A (12-1), 10B (12-2), 11A (13-1), 11B (13-2), 13A (16-1), 13B (16-2), 13C (16-3), 16 (19-1), 17 (21-1), 19A (24-1), 19B (24-2), 19C (24-3), 22 (29-1), 27A (35-1), 27B (35-2), 27C (35-3), 27D (35-4), 29A (37-1), 29B (37-2), 43A (42-1), 43B (42-2), 44 (43-1), 45A (44-1), 45B (44-2), 47 (47-1), 50 (52-1), 51A (53-1), 51B (53-2), 51C (53-3), 52A (55-1), 52B (55-2), 52C (55-3), 53A (56-1), 53B (56-2), 54 (57-1), 55 (59-1), 31A (65-1), 31B (65-2), 31C (65-3), 31D (65-4), 32A (67-1), 32B (67-2), 32C (67-3), 32D (67-4), 33A (68-1), 33B (68-2), 33C (68-3), 34 (69-1), 35 (70-1), 36A (71-1), 36B (71-2), 36C (71-3), 40A (77-1), 40B (77-2), 40C (77-3), 40D (77-4), 41 (78-1), 42 (79-1).

Colman RW et al. *Hemostasis and Thrombosis: Basic Principles and Clinical Practice.* 5th ed. Philadelphia: Lippincott Williams & Wilkins; 2005. Fig. 109-7 (60-1).

Corman ML. *Colon & Rectal Surgery.* 5th ed. Philadelphia: Lippincott Williams & Wilkins; 2004. Fig. 28-26 (76-1).

DeVita VT, Hellman S, Rosenberg SA. *Cancer: Principles and Practice of Oncology.* 7th ed. Philadelphia: Lippincott Williams & Wilkins; 2004. Fig. 43.1-1 (48-1).

Eisenberg RL. *Clinical Imaging: An Atlas of Differential Diagnosis.* 4th ed. Philadelphia: Lippincott Williams & Wilkins; 2002. Figs. CA 20-1 (5-1), GI 55-2 (22-1), B 3-3 (32-1), C 14-4 (58-1), GI 62-1 (62-1), GI 53-1 (63-1), GI 36-10 (66-1).

Feigenbaum H, Armstrong WF, Ryan T. *Feigenbaum's Echocardiography.* 6th ed. Philadelphia: Lippincott Williams & Wilkins; 2004. Fig. 11.22 (17-1).

Gold DH, Weingeist TA. *Color Atlas of the Eye in Systemic Disease.* Baltimore: Lippincott Williams & Wilkins; 2001. Fig. 89.1 (80-1).

Goodheart HP. *Goodheart's Photoguide of Common Skin Disorders.* 2nd ed. Philadelphia: Lippincott Williams & Wilkins; 2003. Fig. 25.8 (30-2).

Greer JP, Foerster J, et al. *Wintrobe's Clinical Hematology.* 11th ed. Philadelphia: Lippincott Williams & Wilkins; 2003. Figs. 38.5 (50-1), 59.3 (51-1).

Humes HD. *Kelley's Textbook of Internal Medicine.* 2nd ed. Philadelphia: Lippincott Williams & Wilkins; 2001. Fig. 411.3 (27-1), Table 399.7 (Table 27-1).

Irwin RS, Rippe JM. *Irwin & Rippe's Intensive Care Medicine.* 5th ed. Philadelphia: Lippincott Williams & Wilkins; 2003. Figs. 104.1 (31-1), 102.5 (36-1).

McClatchey KD et al. *Clinical Laboratory Medicine.* 2nd ed. Philadelphia: Lippincott Williams &Wilkins; 2001. Fig. 44.25c,d (46-1).

Mulholland MW, Lillemoe KD, Doherty GM, et al. *Greenfield's Surgery: Scientific Principles & Practice.* 4th ed. Philadelphia: Lippincott Williams & Wilkins; 2005. Fig. 60.4 (73-1).

Neinstein LS et al. *Adolescent Health Care: A Practical Guide.* 4th ed. Philadelphia: Lippincott Williams & Wilkins. Fig. 31.2 (72-1).

Perrillo RP, Regenstein FG. *Viral and Immune Hepatitis.* In: Kelley WN, ed. *Textbook of Internal Medicine.* 3rd ed. Philadelphia: Lippincott; 1996. Fig. 19.1 (74-2).

Rosen PP. *Rosen's Breast Pathology.* 2nd ed. Philadelphia: Lippincott Williams & Wilkins; 2001. Fig. 14.2a,b (45-1).

Rubin E, Farber JL. *Pathology.* 3rd ed. Philadelphia: Lippincott Williams & Wilkins; 1999. Fig. 14.25 (74-1).

Smeltzer SC, Bare BG. *Brunner & Suddarth's Textbook of Medical-Surgical Nursing.* 9th ed. Philadelphia: Lippincott Williams & Wilkins; 2000. Fig. 35.1 (75-1).

Speroff L, Fritz MA. *Clinical Gynecologic Endocrinology and Infertility.* 7th ed. Philadelphia: Lippincott Williams & Wilkins; 2004. Fig. p. 655 (unnumbered) (38-1).

Topol EJ, Califf RM, Isner J, et al. *Textbook of Cardiovascular Medicine.* 2nd ed. Philadelphia: Lippincott Williams & Wilkins; 2002. Figs. 50.17 (14-1), 60.3 (15-1), 26.3 (18-1), 18.6 (20-1), GU 36-3 (23-1), GU 16-4 (26-1).

Yamada T, Alpers DH, et al. *Textbook of Gastroenterology.* 4th ed. Philadelphia: Lippincott Williams & Wilkins; 2003. Figs. 76-4 (64-1), 76-5 (64-2), 91-3 (66-2), 91-4 (66-3).

# case list

## CARDIOLOGY

1. Acute Bacterial Endocarditis
2. Aortic Insufficiency
3. Aortic Stenosis
4. Atrial Myxoma
5. Cardiac Tamponade
6. Congestive Heart Failure
7. Cor Pulmonale
8. Dilated Cardiomyopathy
9. Hypertensive Urgency
10. Hypertrophic Obstructive Cardiomyopathy
11. Marantic Endocarditis
12. Mitral Insufficiency
13. Mitral Stenosis
14. Myocardial Infarction
15. Paroxysmal Supraventricular Tachycardia
16. Pericarditis
17. Rheumatic Heart Disease
18. Subacute Bacterial Endocarditis
19. Torsades de Pointes
20. Unstable Angina
21. Wolff–Parkinson–White Syndrome

## ENDOCRINOLOGY

22. Addison Disease
23. Conn Syndrome
24. Cushing Disease
25. Diabetes Insipidus
26. Diabetes Mellitus, Type 1
27. Diabetes Mellitus, Type 2
28. Diabetic Ketoacidosis
29. Glucagonoma
30. Graves Disease
31. Hashimoto Thyroiditis
32. Hyperparathyroidism—Primary
33. Hypoparathyroidism
34. Hypothyroidism—Primary
35. Insulinoma
36. Nonketotic Hyperosmolar Coma
37. Osteomalacia
38. Osteoporosis
39. Pheochromocytoma
40. Prolactinoma
41. Syndrome of Inappropriate Secretion of Antidiuretic Hormone (SIADH)

## HEME/ONC

42. Acute Myelogenous Leukemia (AML)
43. Anemia—Iron Deficiency
44. Anemia—Vitamin $B_{12}$ Deficiency
45. Breast Cancer
46. Burkitt Lymphoma
47. Chronic Lymphocytic Leukemia (CLL)
48. Chronic Myelogenous Leukemia (CML)
49. Deep Vein Thrombosis
50. Disseminated Intravascular Coagulation (DIC)
51. Hemophilia A
52. Hereditary Spherocytosis
53. Hodgkin Lymphoma
54. Idiopathic Thrombocytopenic Purpura (ITP)
55. Multiple Myeloma
56. Non-Hodgkin Lymphoma
57. Polycythemia Vera (PCV)
58. Small-Cell Carcinoma of the Lung
59. Thalassemia—Alpha

60. Thrombotic Thrombocytopenic Purpura (TTP)
61. von Willebrand Disease

**GI**
62. Acute Cholecystitis
63. Acute Pancreatitis
64. Celiac Disease
65. Chronic Pancreatitis
66. Colon Cancer
67. Crohn Disease
68. Diverticulosis
69. Gastroesophageal Reflux Disease

70. Hemochromatosis
71. Hepatic Cirrhosis
72. Hepatitis A
73. Hepatitis, Alcoholic
74. Hepatitis B
75. Irritable Bowel Syndrome
76. Ischemic Colitis/Mesenteric Ischemia
77. Peptic Ulcer Disease
78. Primary Biliary Cirrhosis
79. Ulcerative Colitis
80. Wilson Disease

# index